SPEECH REHABILITATION
OF THE
LARYNGECTOMIZED

Publication Number 739
AMERICAN LECTURE SERIES®
A Monograph in
AMERICAN LECTURES IN SPEECH AND HEARING
Edited by
ROBERT WEST
Fellow of the American Speech and Hearing Association
Los Angeles, California

Second Edition, Third Printing

SPEECH REHABILITATION
OF THE
LARYNGECTOMIZED

Compiled and Edited by

JOHN C. SNIDECOR

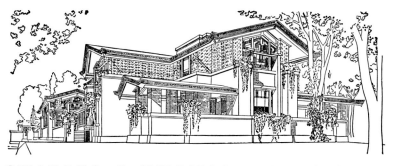

CHARLES C THOMAS · PUBLISHER
Springfield · Illinois · U.S.A.

Published and Distributed Throughout the World by
CHARLES C THOMAS • PUBLISHER
Bannerstone House
301-327 East Lawrence Avenue, Springfield, Illinois, U.S.A.

© *1962 and 1968, by* CHARLES C THOMAS • PUBLISHER

ISBN 0-398-01803-0

Library of Congress Catalog Card Number: 68-9393

First Edition, 1962
Second Edition, 1968
Second Edition, Second Printing, 1974
Second Edition, Third Printing, 1978

With THOMAS BOOKS *careful attention is given to all details of
manufacturing and design. It is the Publisher's desire to present books that
are satisfactory as to their physical qualities and artistic possibilities and
appropriate for their particular use.* THOMAS BOOKS *will be true to those
laws of quality that assure a good name and good will.*

Printed in the United States of America
R-1

Contributors

JOHN C. SNIDECOR, PH.D., F.A.S.H.A.
Professor of Speech
University of California
Santa Barbara, California

JOEL JAY PRESSMAN, M.D., D.SC. (MED.)
Professor of Surgery
Division of Head and Neck Surgery
University of California Medical School
Los Angeles, California

BYRON J. BAILEY, M.D., F.A.A.O.O., F.A.C.S.
Head, Department of Surgery
Head, Department of Surgery/Otolaryngology
Harbor General Hospital
Assistant Professor of Surgery
Division of Head and Neck Surgery
University of California Medical School
Los Angeles, California

ALDEN H. MILLER, M.D.
Clinical Professor and Chairman
Department of Otorhinolaryngology
University of Southern California School of Medicine
Los Angeles, California

EVELYN ROBE FINKBEINER, PH.D.
Former Lecturer in Otolaryngology
Northwestern University Medical School
Research Fellow, William and Harriet Gould Foundation

E. THAYER CURRY, PH.D., F.A.S.H.A.
Professor of Speech
University of Pittsburgh
Pittsburgh, Pennsylvania

ALAN C. NICHOLS, PH.D.
  Associate Professor of Speech
  San Diego State College
  San Diego, California

NOBUHIKO, ISSHIKI, M.D.
  Dozent, School of Medicine,
  University of Kyoto,
  Kyoto, Japan
  Former Assistant Research Laryngologist
  University of California
  Los Angeles, California

JOHN O. ANDERSON, PH.D.
  Professor of Speech and Hearing
  Associate Dean, Graduate School
  Southern Illinois University
  Carbondale, Illinois

Foreword

IN THE LAST twenty years the number of laryngectomees (those whose larynxes have been excised) has steadily increased. The interest of the professional world in those patients has grown correspondingly; and the quality of the rehabilitation of these persons has, as a consequence, markedly improved through extensive research in diagnostic, surgical, and rehabilitative procedures.

The authors of this book give historical perspective to the problem, delve deeply yet economically into research related to it, and develop therapeutic and educational principles and techniques which will be of great assistance to the varied and dedicated practitioners who work with those who would "speak again."

The documentation for both domestic and foreign source materials is the most complete yet assembled, and will benefit the advanced research student and clinician.

In this Second Edition the original chapters have been brought up-to-date, and many new facets of the subject have been presented. Results of recent airflow studies by Drs. Snidecor and Isshiki have been incorporated and interpreted. Dr. Alden H. Miller discusses techniques of the new Asai laryngoplasty operation. Professor Snidecor, the senior author, traveled to Japan where he served as Visiting Professor at the University of Kyoto. There and at the University of Kobe he studied Asai speech at first hand. The senior author also added over 300 items to the 546 bibliographic items presented in the edition of 1962.

ROBERT WEST
Editor

Preface

THIS BOOK IS written for the research-oriented practitioner who deals with the medical, psychological, and educational problems of those individuals who must lose, or who have already lost, all or a significant portion of the larynx. The approach leads through history and research to practice, but with definite, built-in limitations. For example, the chapter by Joel J. Pressman and Byron J. Bailey emphasizes the partial laryngectomy with the assumption that most interested surgeons will already be completely familiar with total extirpation. The senior author, when writing about speech therapy, has attempted to avoid the "cookbook" approach and instead to define principles from which drill materials have been derived with the thought that this approach enables the clinician to produce a variety of new drill materials.

The laryngectomee is dealt with directly in Chapters XI through XV and he as a patient might profit from reading these chapters in particular. However, in case he should experience a kind of semantic indigestion, it is suggested that he have a session or two with the speech clinician before this assignment takes place.

The advanced graduate student may be assigned the entire book, and to him we invite special attention to Chapters I through X for here lies the bulk of the research materials which contribute to "doctor's orals" and backgrounds for insightful practice.

Acknowledgments in this book are dealt with almost exclusively within the text and the substantial Bibliography and References. The special acknowledgments stated below are those that do not quite fit the rubrics of editorial design.

Our first special acknowledgment is to all of the generous laryngectomees who participated in the research that made this book possible. Of those who have learned to speak again and are extensively quoted, we mention with emphasis Joe Green, the late Laurance Phelps, and the late Hiram Hall.

Teachers and colleagues who should be mentioned here are the late Grant Fairbanks who, as a former teacher, influenced the experimental design and procedures in Chapters V and VI, and the nature of the drills in Chapters XIII and XIV; and Robert Harrington whose constructive criticism helped significantly in the final formulation of the chapters on speech therapy. Bernard Stoll's materials helped greatly in the discussion of personal factors; Henry J. Rubin's ultra high-speed photographs, taken under the auspices of U.S.P.H.S., clarified written materials in Chapter IV. Without the surgical skill of Dr. Asai, there would have been no reason to write Chapter VIII, nor could it have been accomplished without the collaboration of Drs. Isshiki and Kimura, and the assistance of Drs. Honjow and Okamura. Because Dr. Anderson was not available, the author leaned heavily on the help of Mrs. Verniece Narkis for the Bibliography. Finally, the patient and effective editorial work of my wife, Lois E. Snidecor, has contributed greatly to uniformity of style and precision of statement.

We are indebted to many publishers and publishing houses, and especially to the following: E. and S. Livingstone, Ltd., of Edinburgh for case studies from *Speech Recovery After Total Laryngectomy* by Hodson and Oswald; *Laryngoscope* for materials in Chapter IV and elsewhere; *Annals of Otology, Rhinogology* and *Laryngology,* especially for the materials in Chapter III; *Speech Monographs* for materials in Chapter V; *Acta Oto-Laryngology* for materials in Chapter IX; *Folia Phoniatrica* for materials in Chapter X. Two plates in Chapter II are presented with the permission of Masson & Cié., Paris.

J. C. S.

Contents

SPEECH REHABILITATION
OF THE
LARYNGECTOMIZED

Chapter I

The Nature of the Problem

John C. Snidecor

Historical Notes

FOR THOUSANDS of years, man died as a result of cancer of the larynx and because of other laryngeal disorders and injuries. Today, the well-informed layman has some knowledge of the importance of the larynx in terms of its functions as a valve to protect the lungs and as a means of communication, but he is not always well enough informed to save his life or at best his voice from the ravages of cancer. We use the term *he* on purpose, for approximately ten men to one woman will have cancer of the larynx.

Until Antyllus (823), in about A.D., 120 performed what was probably the first tracheotomy, there was not even temporary relief from the gradual stoppage of air which often accompanied cancerous growth within the larynx. In case one might exaggerate the number and importance of early tracheotomies, it should be noted that Richter (823) invented the modern tracheotomy tube at the time of our Revolutionary War, and it was a few years later that tracheotomy was reported as performed by Andree for croupous laryngitis.

The larynx was a black box defying internal examination in living man until Worden, Avery, and especially Manuel Garcia (459) developed the laryngoscope which was so simple in concept and so essential to modern laryngology.

Garcia's publication came in 1855 and, although he was only one of the independent discoverers of the laryngoscope, he gave the instrument the attention it deserved throughout his long professional life. He died in 1906 (at the age of 102), having been honored on the occasion of his centenary by laryngologists who came from all over the world to do him honor in London. Although laryngectomy was and is primarily external, the initial internal examination depends upon Garcia's bright light and round mirror.

The first laryngectomy for cancer was performed by Billroth (459) in 1873, although a previous total extirpation had been performed a few years before by Watson for a syphilitic infection. Within six years from the time of Billroth's operation, at least nineteen laryngectomies had been accomplished and reported. The rate of success by modern standards was not high, but improved rapidly, and by 1890 at least two-hundred laryngectomies had been performed.

In 1967, according to the American Cancer Society, there are 3,000 surviving laryngectomees added each year to the approximately 23,000 total laryngectomees alive in the United States. Within the last ten years, according to the National Cancer Institute, there has been a 75 per cent increase in cancer of the larynx with, however, only a 42 per cent increase in mortality. Certainly the total incidence is approximately 4 in 100,000 of the general population.

The introductory historical comments discussed briefly above will be somewhat expanded in various chapters. It is now desirable to turn to the nature of the problem as a personal experience.

The Man and the Operation

It is, after all, a *man* who has cancer of the larynx. He may be an essential surgical and historical statistic to others, but he is much more to himself and his family.

Hiram Hall was an investment banker who retired in Santa Barbara. He died only recently of causes other than cancer. As a friend of the author, he spoke and later wrote this story:

> The verdict was cancer. The biopsy was the final proof of that. My doctor had tried to prepare me, but I had refused to believe that this could happen to me. Mercifully the shock was so terrific, of course, as to be numbing. The doctor briefed me on the necessary operation and on what I might expect afterward. My voice box would be removed so that I could no longer speak by old methods. I must develop a new voice, a difficult but quite possible thing to do.
>
> An immediate operation was arranged for and performed, and I

found myself in my hospital bed bristling with tubes from mouth and nostrils and with a new opening about the size of a five cent piece in my throat. This opening connected with the windpipe and was to be my way of breathing thereafter. My nose would be of little use except to hold my glasses on. I cannot say I was happy or comfortable, though I tried to appear so to nurses and my family and doctors who all tried to cheer me and encourage. The frustration caused by inability to communicate is intense. All my remarks or answers to questions had to be written on a pad. My writing is not too legible at best.

My family shed no tears in public, but their gaiety sometimes seemed to be forced. During those long days in bed, I made a deep resolve to learn to speak. At last I was at home once more. And I was often alone. I spent the long hours on the patio striving to make sounds by the gulp and burp method about which my doctor had told me. I had no instructor and had never heard a laryngectomee speak, and at first no sound other than a burp would come. But slowly, painfully, I succeeded. The first real word I uttered was beautiful in my ears. It was "no," and it amazed and delighted my son to whom I said it.

After that, my new voice developed rapidly — from one-syllable words to two, then three. Sentences followed, and at last I would converse in a voice hoarse, but to me wonderful. I could abandon the pad and pencil and the sign language. And what a relief it was. My prayers had been answered — prayers often repeated. Of course, prayer has to be backed up by a deep desire to speak. You must give it all you have, and never quit trying. After the first word, it comes easier.

Adjustment to the new way of life is not easy, but it can be achieved. Life goes on; there is still happiness in store.

Here I will mention a few things which are lost to the laryngectomee. The sense of smell is limited, and with it taste is diminished. I cannot laugh aloud, although I still laugh silently. I can whistle, however, and I'm quite proud of that.

When a learned doctor of the University of California who had been making a study of the speech of laryngectomees declared my voice one of the best of about fifty tested, I was indeed gratified.

When Joe Green, veteran *Cincinnati Inquirer* reporter, had his laryngectomy he wrote a series of articles for his own and other newspapers. The following long quotation is from the *Santa Barbara News-Press*, March 13, 1960 and at the expense of some slight repetition describes the nature of the experience and the operation in straightforward descriptive terms. Green's statement in regard to surgery is clarified in Figures 1 and 2. Figure 3 details the new Asai operation. See Chapter VIII.

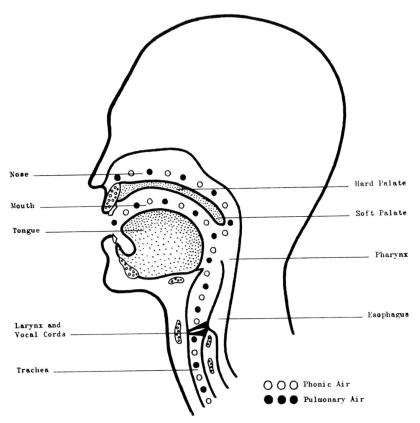

Nose

Mouth

Tongue

Larynx and
Vocal Cords

Trachea

Hard Palate

Soft Palate

Pharynx

Esophagus

O O O Phonic Air
● ● ● Pulmonary Air

FIGURE 1. The head and neck before total laryngectomy.

CINCINNATI (AP)—When the doctor told me I had cancer of the vocal chords I was more shocked than surprised.

Now I realized that I had suspected it all along.

The doctor looked at a sheet of paper on which was typewritten a long paragraph. It was a pathologist's report of a biopsy made three days before at St. Elizabeth Hospital in Covington, Ky.

"It showed 'positive' this time; I'm sorry," he said. "We have been worried about it from the very first."

That was last July 26. Five months before, my vocal chords had been "stripped" for a first biopsy. The report then was "negative." But my luck hadn't held.

"We've talked over this possibility before," the doctor went on. "Two things can be done. One is surgery; the other is x-ray treatments.

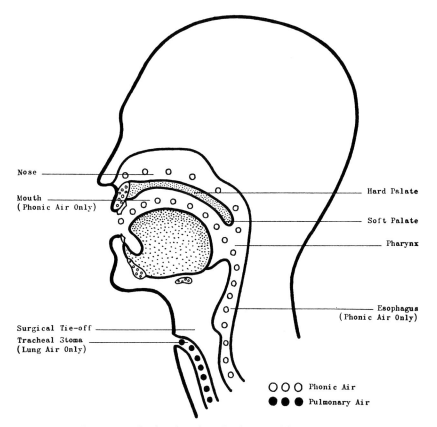

Nose

Mouth
(Phonic Air Only)

Surgical Tie-off

Tracheal Stoma
(Lung Air Only)

Hard Palate

Soft Palate

Pharynx

Esophagus
(Phonic Air Only)

O O O Phonic Air
● ● ● Pulmonary Air

FIGURE 2. The head and neck after total laryngectomy.

"Surgery seems to us to be the sure way. We excise the tumor by removing the entire larynx and the vocal cords."

He didn't mention the "do nothing about it" alternative — long suffering and death after a year or so. It took no great amount of courage to choose surgery.

It had all started a few weeks before Christmas, 1958. I developed hoarseness which no amount of medication would clear up, and at times I couldn't speak above a whisper.

When the hoarseness persisted, the first biopsy was made. Even after the negative finding, the throat condition, complicated by a nose infection, did not clear up entirely. I couldn't trust my voice to function when I needed it.

Four weeks in Florida did wonders. I went back to work in May.

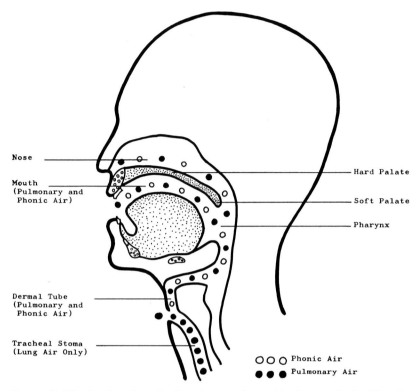

FIGURE 3. The head and neck after laryngoplasty (Asai operation). The size of the dermal tube is exaggerated to show the direction of airflow.

My elation was short-lived. Constant use of my voice in telephone conversations, in interviews, and in day-to-day associations battered the vocal cords. On July 18 they just conked out.

"You will have to give up something. Cases like this always call for sacrifice."

The doctor was telling me I would have to surrender my speech.

"Through speech therapy you will learn to talk again — almost as good as you do now," the doctor said. "Maybe your voice will be a little deeper, and you'll never sing in the opera, but you'll talk.

"I want to warn you, however, it will be no easy job. It probably will be the most frustrating and aggravating task you ever faced and it will take a long time to master it."

Then I received a briefing:

"The larynx will be removed and the air that once passed through your throat from the lungs will be sealed off by surgery so it will pass in and out of an opening at the neck, right there. (The doctor placed a finger to a spot just above my breastbone.)

"This entrance will supply the body with oxygen; the air you breathe will have no value in production of speech."

"But, how will I blow my nose?" I wanted to know.

With no pressure from the lungs available, a sufferer from nose infections, hay fever, or even a cold would face complications.

The doctor had no quick answer.

"I hadn't thought of it," he grinned. "It's a good question, though. I guess you just wipe your nose."

He set the operation for Aug. 6 — nine days away.

Late the afternoon of Aug. 5, the surgeon sat on a side of my hospital bed and talked calmly of the operation he would perform next day.

"There was a time when a total laryngectomy was unheard of, and many people died from cancer of the vocal cords," he explained to me and my wife. "It's done all the time now . . . .

"You should be up and out of here in 10 days or two weeks."

Then he left. My wife went home.

There's something dreadfully lonesome about a hospital room just before dusk, when the dinner is over, the visitors have gone and a long night approaches.

I sat there a long time. It wasn't fear I felt. I just hated it. There was no alternative. I was resigned to surgery, having consoled myself that the tumor had been found in time . . . .

During the weeks of recuperation, the curious and interested beset me with numerous questions: "How can you eat?" "Can you taste?" "How come you are smoking again?"

Here are some of the answers:

Normally, both food and air follow a common passage before they hit a fork in the road — then they take separate ways. This passage is called the pharynx and begins at the base of the tongue. At its lower end the food turns into one of the forks — the esophagus — and the air turns into the other — the larynx.

When the larynx is removed by surgery, the windpipe is severed and bent forward to the neck where it is sutured to the opening made just above the breastbone. Through this opening, the laryngectomee must breathe. It leads directly into the windpipe. When a laryngectomee sneezes or coughs, he holds his handkerchief to this opening — not to the mouth and nose. When he gets accustomed to it, that is.

After the surgeon removes the larynx, he ties off the space it occupied, setting up a wall between the windpipe and the esophagus. When the wall is healed, the patient can eat whatever he chooses — and taste it, too.

As for smoking — a habit banned in my case before the biopsy detected cancer — it can do no harm now, the doctors say. The smoke does not enter the throat or lungs.

That's why I resumed pipe smoking.

Who Helps

It is impossible to list all of the organizations, let alone individuals, that have helped and are helping in determined efforts to further medical, social, educational, and economic attacks on cancer.

The first great surgical breakthrough came almost one hundred years ago with the work of such men as Billroth, Maas, Bottini, and Rubio (459) who first operated and then meticulously recorded their results in medical journals, and often in personal communications to each other. Throughout the years, interest in surgery and related problems has grown. Operations have often been perfected on animals, and then on man. Since the turn of the century, x-ray treatments have been utilized.

Closely related to the medical approach per se are biomedical and biochemical studies which, through basic research, discover heredogenetic, physiological, and chemical relationships for states of health and disease. Only very recently, carcinomic tissue has been grown in test tubes. When the breakthrough comes, it may well be through basic laboratory research.

A very special kind of study has gone into the artificial larynx which is as old as the laryngectomy. To be sure, no dramatic developments in intelligibility have been made, but some improvement is in evidence, and the instrument has become more attractive, convenient, and in the case of the electric larynx, more economical to operate. It should be noted that even today some countries, especially Spain and Japan, favor the artificial larynx over esophageal speech. Progress in esophageal speech instruction is being made in both of these countries. For those who favor the old air-driven Western Electric Larynx, it will be of interest that the author purchased an air-driven larynx in Japan for six dollars and fifty cents. The construction is simple and intelligibility is good.

The social and educational aspects of cancer of the larynx can be discussed together, for they are closely related. No single group is doing more for this two-sided problem than the International Association of Laryngectomees (IAL), which is an autonomous agency supported by the American Cancer Society.

It is easy to understand why those who have been deprived of speech might seek social isolation. Executive Secretary of IAL, Jack L. Ranney, expresses it this way: "One of our big jobs is to find them and get them to the speech centers. . . . Sometimes we find a man who perhaps hasn't said a word in ten years. You can imagine what it means to him and his family to be able to talk again. Often it is the difference between holding or getting a job or being permanently unemployed."

Rehabilitation begins before the operation and continues until the individual is speaking and back on the job or, if retired, speaking and back to normal family and social relationships.

IAL was conceived by Warren H. Gardner, Ph.D., of the Cleveland Hearing and Speech Clinic in 1951. In 1953, IAL was organized through assistance from the American Cancer Society. The assistance of the parent society continues.

Local *Lost Chord Clubs* and *New Voice Clubs* are now frequently affiliated with IAL, but they continue their local autonomy and service to laryngectomees. The international aspects of the program were developed in large part through the efforts of the late Edmund C. Johnson who was not only instrumental in founding the Lost Chord Club of Southern California but who went on, at his own expense, to travel around the world and develop interest in and understanding of IAL. In the last nine or ten years, IAL has been especially active on the international scene and has developed 134 affiliated clubs which have contact with more than 12,000 laryngectomees. The *IAL News* is a bimonthly, distributed free of charge, and now goes to more than 18,000 persons, including those in fifty-five countries. IAL is both an important and large organization within the United States. As of 1968, there are approximately 125 clubs with a total membership of approximately 15,000.

No introductory statement about IAL would be complete without mentioning, in addition to the names already stated, Mrs. Mary Doehler, a seventy-six-year-old grandmother, who has been an officer in IAL until recently and who has taught over 1,200 laryngectomees. She will be remembered as the subject for a 1959 article in the *Reader's Digest* entitled "The Irritating Angel." Also, William Gargan, American actor, has been active in presenting the case for the laryngectomee on radio and television and has participated in many conferences throughout the country. John Hawkins, British actor and laryngectomee, has served a similar function in England.

Among the agencies in speech research, therapy, and education is the American Speech and Hearing Association (9030 Old Georgetown Road, Washington, D. C. 20014) which has rigorous standards for full membership and certification. Through its members and journals, information is disseminated concerning all types of speech and hearing problems. A booklet listing those especially qualified to teach esophageal speech is published by the association. In September of 1946, the *Journal of Speech Disorders,* which was at that time the official journal of the organization, contained as lead article "Speech After Laryngectomy" by Bangs, Lierle, and Strother. This brief six-page article presented in an accurate and precise manner the practical knowledge then available concerning esophageal speech and the artificial larynx. The impact of the article was significant because of its availability and practicality and because it came at a time when the laryngectomy operation was becoming much more frequent. Since World War II, the annual increase in incidence of the operation is about 4 per cent.

Medical, social, and speech-educational attacks on cancer would not be possible without appropriate economic support. It is traditional in this country that the private patient pay or prepay the costs of his own medical care when he is able to do so. However, it is as impossible and unrealistic to expect the patient to pay through fees for medical research as it is to expect the practicing physician to do extensive research within the confines of private practice. The plagues of tuberculosis and poliomyelitis have come under control because large private associations have collected and effectively utilized the small contributions of many which, when combined, have amounted to millions of dollars.

Public funds have helped. The American Cancer Society is a voluntary health agency that supports research, education, and community service, but which cannot bear the entire burden of the costs of medical research on cancer.

In 1967, almost a billion dollars was spent on medical research. Approximately half of this money came from private sources and approximately half of it from government sources. The figures, of course, are only estimates because of the large amount of money spent regionally and locally which is not always reported to any national agency.

How One Helps Himself

The American Cancer Society states that the danger signals of cancer should be heeded and medical attention sought if one or more signals persist for longer than two weeks. Among the danger signals for laryngeal cancer are hoarseness, difficulty in swallowing, bleeding, coughing, and soreness. The signals *need not be accompanied by pain.*

Regular health checkups supplemented by special examinations when these are indicated are obvious precautionary measures. Early recognition and treatment in cancer of the larynx may mean only subtotal laryngectomy or may insure the success of total laryngectomy. The examination for laryngeal cancer is normally made by a specialized physician in his own office or at a medical center. It behooves the patient to get competent advice and follow it promptly. Even inside medical practice, and more frequently outside of it, there are quacks who promise cures by methods acceptable to the patient, whereas in reality the only hope is through difficult and prompt decisions followed by prompt action. By way of example, a patient might have been told by competent authority that his total larynx should be promptly removed, and then he might receive the lethal and criminal advice from another source that he could be cured by "magical rays," or "radioactive lozenges."

What has been said, briefly, is that it is the responsibility of the individual layman to be intelligent and courageous in seeking appropriate medical counsel and in following the counsel with promptness.

To smoke or not to smoke has been a private decision based often upon psychological factors of long standing. Until recently, there have been few if any organizations taking a formal and rational stand in regard to smoking. Lack of evidence has limited the quality of scientific and medical advice.

As recently as 1960, the American Cancer Society came out with statistics and statements indicating that the organization took the stand that smoking and cancer are related. There are, of course, other factors, especially city smoke and "smog." To do everything possible to escape cancer of the respiratory tract, one should live in clean country air and abstain from smoking. Such a life is often impractical or even undesirable, and so extra care with precautionary examinations is in order for those who live in or create their own contaminated air. A famous surgeon said recently, "All laryngectomies could be subtotals if the cancer could always be detected early enough."

Recent opinion states that if the case against the safety of the Brooklyn Bridge was as tight as the case against the safety of smoking, it would be closed to traffic at once.

Only a few years ago, the conventions of those who deal with the human throat (medical and educational specialists) were held in the traditional smoke-filled rooms. This is no longer the case, for a very substantial number of these specialists have quit smoking — and breaking the habit of smoking is a trying and time-extended experience as many can testify. In fairness, it must be stated that some persons quit, for example, because they are allergic to tobacco, and others because of heart problems.

The case against smoking is not based on all of the tenets of the professional logician or statistician, but the corelationship of cancer and smoke-laden air, especially for the male of the species, is sufficient proof for many. The burden of proof has shifted to those who claim that smoking is harmless.

It must be stressed that both pulmonary and laryngeal cancer have been under consideration. Drastic and dramatic as laryngeal cancer is, its victims are relatively few compared with those of lung cancer.

Speech Therapy

No introductory chapter would be complete without a brief note concerning speech therapy. It will have been noted that Hiram Hall, whose case was presented earlier, had no speech therapy and had not even heard of a laryngectomee. Mr. Hall learned under difficulties. Joe Green, on the other hand, received direct instruction, and his learning was easier and probably consumed less time. Before and after a laryngectomy, and when released for speech therapy by the surgeon, the patient should see a competent speech therapist. The bases for this choice are discussed in Chapter XII.

Chapter II

The Surgery of Cancer of the Larynx with Especial Reference to Subtotal Laryngectomy

JOEL JAY PRESSMAN AND BYRON J. BAILEY

Introduction

FOR THE PHONETICIST, the surgery of cancer of the larynx resolves itself into the problem of residual speech following the operation. The surgeon, on the other hand, while not at all unmindful of his responsibilities in this direction, is primarily concerned with effecting a cure of the disease.

The two points of view are by no means incompatible. Many types of operations are now available to bring these two closer together. These range from simple direct laryngoscopic removal of small tumors with essentially no postoperative disability, to wide subtotal resections leaving only small fractions of the larynx intact which the surgeon hopefully utilizes for reconstruction in an effort to reestablish a lumen adequate for sound production, even if not for breathing.

As a general rule, it can be stated that the lesser the degree of residual speech anticipated following removal of any given lesion, the greater is the likelihood of surgical cure. In other words, if every surgically operable case of cancer of the larynx were to be treated by extensive total laryngectomy destroying the voice instead of a less radical procedure, the cure rate of this disease would reach the maximum. But if this were done, of course, a great many patients who could survive with less extensive surgery and still retain a useful voice would unnecessarily be laryngectomized.

By having effectively developed the technique of esophageal speech, the speech therapist has greatly lessened the degree of disability incidental to total removal of the larynx.

On the other hand, progress in speech rehabilitation has not relieved the surgeon of his responsibility to continue to develop surgical techniques with as little destruction as possible, commensurate with reasonable safety. The surgeon, in developing new operations and methods of treatment, has attempted to close the gap between doing too little in the interest of voice at the possible risk of life, and too much in the interest of the cure rate at the expense of sacrifice of the patient's ability to phonate. Thus there has come into being a number of new surgical techniques in the nature of partial or subtotal laryngectomies designed to lessen the hazard of the more conservative procedures, and yet yield the maximum result in voice production.

As we learn more and more about the details of the route of spread of this disease, its natural history, the relative resistance of certain tissues to cancer and the greater susceptibility of others, the various details pertaining to tissue spaces, lymphatic flow, and other basic problems concerned, the more intelligently we can cope with the problem of each patient as an individual rather than as a member of a statistical group. The ultimate goal of the surgeon therefore is to provide the best voice possible without undue jeopardy to life.

Great strides forward have been made in this direction, and today the patient with cancer of the larynx — recognized early — enjoys an excellent chance of cure while retaining a good residual voice.

The first operation designed with this thought in mind was "thyrotomy," or splitting the thyroid cartilage at its angle in order to gain access to its interior. The basic technique was introduced by Brauers (86) in 1833 for the treatment of laryngeal polyps. It is now commonly called "laryngofissure." Ehrmann (193), eleven years later, used this technique in the first recorded attempt to cure cancer of the larynx surgically. The effort unfortunately failed. The first known surgical cure of cancer of the larynx was nevertheless accomplished by using this method, J. Solis-Cohen (713) having reported a successful single case in 1868. The earliest reported series of such operations was by P. Bruns (99), who in 1878 presented fifteen patients — all of whom rapidly developed recurrences except one patient who died of intercurrent disease.

Over the years — as surgical techniques, anesthesia, and postoperative care improved, and our knowledge of the natural history of the disease increased — a great many surgical cures in properly selected cases resulted from the use of Brauers' techniques of laryngofissure. The bibliography pertaining to this has become enormous, but certainly none have done more to perfect and popularize the method than Chevalier Jackson and his son, Chevalier L. Jackson (359). Their introduction of the "anterior commissure" operation, by which extensions near or beyond the midline are adequately resected, greatly widened the scope of this technique. However, thyrotomy and resection of a segment of vocal cord can be performed only in cases of limited extent and with the disease confined to the vocal cords. X-ray therapy has advanced sufficiently to provide an equally high rate of cure in cases of such distribution (90 % or more), and this latter method of treatment is therefore often used instead of surgical removal by laryngofissure.

The first total laryngectomy was performed in 1866 by Watson (800) of Edinburg, not for cancer of the larynx but for syphilis. Seven years later, Billroth (75) reported the first total extirpation of the larynx for cancer, the patient surviving the operation but dying of recurrence of cancer eight months later.

The early prohibitive mortality of total laryngectomy, principally from intercurrent infection, encouraged Gluck (270) to attempt a two-stage approach in which the trachea was first severed and sewn to the skin, thus completing the first stage. The larynx was removed later when healing took place. Gluck's procedure fell short of expectations and was rapidly abandoned even by Gluck himself, but it contributed one great advance: the suturing of the severed tracheal stump to the skin margin to form a tracheal stoma in the neck just above the sternum. This became the standard procedure and has been used ever since.

George Crile (138) of Cleveland, recognizing certain possible advantages of total extirpation of the larynx in stages, modified Gluck's concept and instead of severing the trachea as a first step, skeletonized the larynx and trachea, packing gauze around it to produce adhesions which isolated the surgical area from the mediastinum, and after these had formed, removing the larynx in a second stage. This greatly lessened the likelihood of post-operative infection in the chest cavity.

In 1876, ten years after Watson's first total laryngectomy, Maas (457) of Breslau introduced an operation more extensive than laryngofissure for cases limited to one side but not confined to the vocal cord alone. By his method, a portion of the larynx was removed; the residual fraction was preserved and, with some reconstruction, continued to serve as a respiratory airway via normal channels, as well as a source of sound for the production of a whisper, which the patient preferred to the use of Billroth's artificial larynx with which he had been supplied.

A modification of this "subtotal laryngectomy" known as "hemilaryngectomy" or the removal of a lateral half of the larynx was first reported by Billroth (75) of Vienna about two years later. This procedure, being relatively easy to perform and accompanied by a much lower operative mortality than total removal of the larynx, initially enjoyed great popularity. However, after the initial enthusiasm for its use had given way to disappointment, hemilaryngectomy was abandoned. The mortality, though lower than for total laryngectomy, was nevertheless too high for the relatively low cure rate which resulted. Periodically, however, this operation has, since Billroth first introduced it, been revived. There seems little doubt that its initial failure had been due to improper selection of cases resulting from lack of knowledge of the natural history of the disease and from inadequacies in the details of surgical technique. In 1930, however, Marcel Ombré-danne (555) of L'Hospital Tenon et de L'Institute Curie published a monograph describing a series of hemilaryngectomies performed by the technique of A. Hautant (314) and, while the method has not gained general recognition, it overcame many objections applicable to previous techniques and is to be highly recommended. More will be said about it later.

The advantages of any method of successful subtotal removal of involved portions of the larynx as opposed to total removal are obvious. The airway, even in those instances in which it will not suffice for normal respiration, is adequate for phonation via normal channels, so that there is no need for esophageal speech.

The success of subtotal laryngectomy, insofar as the cure rate is concerned, depends upon the proper selection of cases, ordinarily those in which the tumor has not extended beyond the confines of the larynx. This is not always easy to determine preoperatively. There is, therefore, a decided advantage in the use of any surgical method which exposes both sides of the deeper structures of the neck and permits the surgeon to determine, by visual observation and palpation at surgery, the presence or absence of extension into the neighboring tissue spaces or into the lymph nodes of the neck. The nodes are part of the lymphatic chain accompanying the great vessels of the neck, the carotid arteries, and internal jugular veins. Because of thick overlying muscles, such nodes are not always palpable by direct preoperative examination.

The method, widely exposing the larynx and contiguous areas of the neck for subtotal laryngectomies, accounts in no small measure for the success of recent techniques which permit visualization of the more likely areas of spread beyond the larynx. This is in contrast to the use of small incisions of limited extent which overlie just the midline of the larynx itself. Furthermore, techniques which take the larynx apart in the process of removal, rather than consisting of a blind en bloc resection as is the case in the standard hemilaryngectomy, provide the surgeon with an opportunity to determine if spread beyond the confines of the larynx is imminent, in which case a total laryngectomy had better be performed.

The decision as to whether to perform a total laryngectomy with permanent loss of the normal voice, or a partial laryngectomy which preserves the normal airway for purposes of speech, cannot always be decided by the size of the cancer within the larynx. The fact that the tumor appears large to the examiner can be misleading in that its base, from which extension into the deeper tissues takes place, may be very small, with a pedunculated or mushroom-like pattern of growth, the stem representing the site of origin. Other tumors, especially those arising in the ventricle of the larynx which appear very small to the examiner, may have spread fan-like between the soft structures of the interior of the larynx and the cartilaginous walls, or even beyond the confines of the larynx into tissues of the neck and yet present, by visual mirror examination of the larynx, only a very small lesion indeed.

While x-ray examination by tomography may give good evidence of the extent of such lesions, it is not to be depended upon entirely, and the final decision as to what to do from the surgical standpoint can, with assurance, be made only at the operating table with the structures exposed to direct view. It follows, therefore, as a general rule, that any partial or subtotal laryngectomy which takes the larynx apart and thereby permits evaluation of the extent of the lesion can be relied upon to give better results than en bloc resections which do not. The development of the newer surgical techniques is now based on sound fundamental basic laboratory experiments.

Recently gained knowledge concerning the anatomy of the spread of cancer within the larynx and its route of escape beyond, into the structures of the neck, has contributed enormously to the successful treatment of this disease by permitting the use of conservative surgical techniques which preserve the normal functions of speech and respiration in a far greater number of cases than was true even a decade ago. These current experiments, upon which our knowledge of the natural history of this disease has been advanced, have been conducted on dogs, pigs, and the human living and cadiver larynx, and the findings have been correlated with observations upon numerous laryngeal specimens surgically removed at various clinics as well as with autopsy findings. From these studies, certain conclusions are now considered justified.

1. The interior of the larynx is divided into a number of compartments which are more or less isolated from one another insofar as communication by direct spread or the lymphatics between them is concerned. The early spread of cancer within the confines of each compartment is to be expected by reason of lessened resistance to the direction of growth; but spread from one compartment to the next is long delayed by reason of the resistance offered by these tissue boundaries. Such compartmentation can be demonstrated by the injection of dyes into the cadaver larynx. Generally speaking, the compartments consist of one

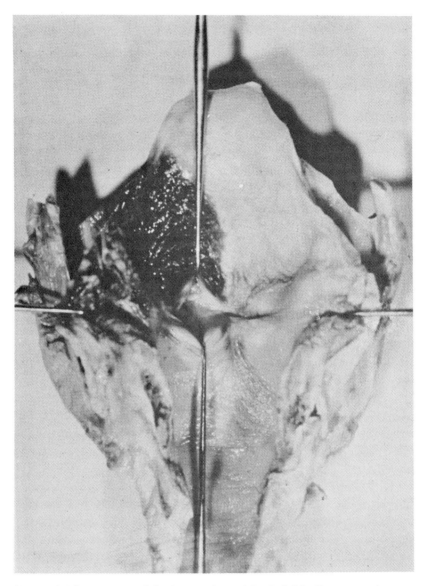

FIGURE 4. Tissue spaces of the larynx (aryepiglottic fold). Demonstrating one of the "tissue spaces" of the larynx. The supraglottic space is filled with dye injected under pressure. The interior of the ventricle is exposed to show that dye has not invaded it. Notice failure of dye to cross the midline.

located below the true vocal cord; the margin of the true vocal cord; the ventricle itself; the area above the ventricle including the false vocal cord and the aryepiglottic fold; and finally the cartilaginous epiglottis. The margin of the true vocal cord is formed by a bursal sac which seems to be even more isolated from the remainder of the larynx than any of the others. As a result, tumors limited to this area have an excellent prognosis if properly treated, and the cure rate is very high.

2. The lymphatic flow within the boundaries of the larynx represents a second route of spread of laryngeal cancer (the first being by direct spread) . This flow is always upward, beginning at the level of the lower border of the cricoid cartilage. The clinical significance of this from the standpoint of the surgical cure of cancer of the larynx is not to be underestimated. Lesions extending below the level of the cricoid cartilage ordinarily require a much more guarded prognosis and far wider excisions than those not so situated.

3. From the standpoint of spread from one side of the larynx to the other, one needs to consider the mucous membrane as being entirely independent of the deeper structures. The former evidently develops embryologically as a single sheet, which spreads across the larynx from one side to the other, carrying the lymphatic network freely across the midline. This suggests the likelihood of superficial malignant tumors spreading readily from one side to the other, and this is borne out by clinical observation. The deeper structures, however, as represented by the compartments of the larynx, do not readily communicate from one side to the other. This can be demonstrated by the deep injection of dyes or radioisotopes which, when so injected into one side of the living dog or human larynx, remain confined to that one side for many weeks or months, even though spread into the general lymphatic circulation of the body takes place immediately upon injection, and the presence of such substances, particularly the radioisotopes, can be identified almost immediately in various organs of the body.

This peculiar situation, in which one lateral half of the larynx is isolated from the other, can be explained upon the basis of its embryonic development. Each half of the thyroid cartilage, and the muscles attached to it, develops independently as a separate structure. Fusion of the two halves to form one single organ takes place through the medium of a third little-known and seldom-described embryonic structure. This is a narrow midline strip of fetal cartilage called the "intralaryngeal cartilage," which ultimately loses its identity. By reason of fusion, independently to the intralaryngeal cartilage, the two halves of the larynx form a single organ. However, this fusion, taking place in later embryonic life after the lymphatics have formed, does not permit an inter-

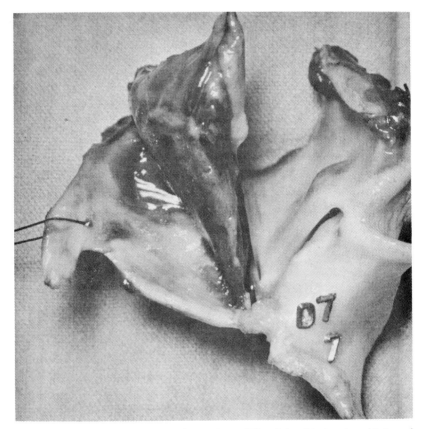

FIGURE 5. Interior of dog larynx from above. The right side has been injected with dye seven hours prior to sacrifice. Note failure of dye to be carried across the midline either by direct extension or lymphatic spread.

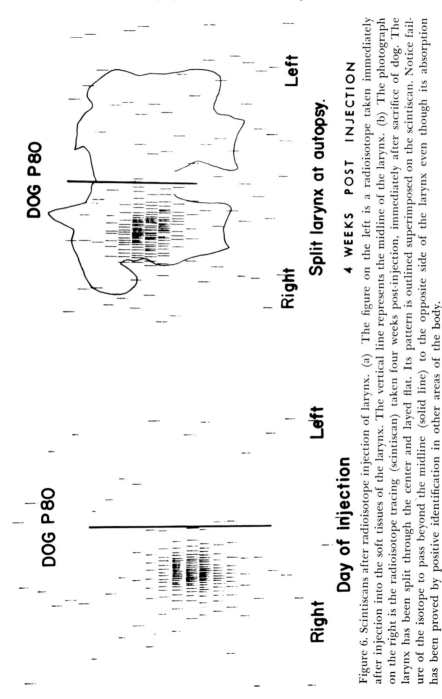

Figure 6. Scintiscans after radioisotope injection of larynx. (a) The figure on the left is a radioisotope taken immediately after injection into the soft tissues of the larynx. The vertical line represents the midline of the larynx. (b) The photograph on the right is the radioisotope tracing (scintiscan) taken four weeks post-injection, immediately after sacrifice of dog. The larynx has been split through the center and layed flat. Its pattern is outlined superimposed on the scintiscan. Notice failure of the isotope to pass beyond the midline (solid line) to the opposite side of the larynx even though its absorption has been proved by positive identification in other areas of the body.

mingling of the deeper lymphatics of one side with those of the other, or the joining of the submucosal laryngeal compartments of one side to those of the other. This accounts for the physiological and anatomical isolation, except for the mucous membrane of one lateral half of the larynx from the other, and explains in large measure the clinical behaviors of many cancers of the larynx. Knowledge of these details permits the decision concerning the type of operation to be performed in any given case to be based upon fundamental facts and largely eliminates the factor of guesswork. It is this approach to the problem which has improved the cure rate and at the same time has diminished the number of patients requiring the use of esophageal speech.

Total Laryngectomy

The best known operation related to the surgical treatment of cancer of the larynx is total laryngectomy, which removes en bloc both true and false vocal cords, the ventricles, the arytenoid cartilages, the epiglottis, and the cricoid cartilage. The hyoid bone is usually but not always included. The attached extrinsic muscles coming from the sternum to the larynx and from the larynx to the bone are usually included.

Often times, when spread beyond the lymphatics to the lymph nodes of the neck is proven or even strongly suspected, all removable structures of the involved side of the neck or even both sides are included, which procedure is known as the "radical neck dissection." When performed together with total laryngectomy, one describes the operation as "total laryngectomy with radical neck dissection in continuity." Thus, in addition to the larynx and attached ribbon muscles, there is removed the sternocleidomastoid and omohyoid muscles, the muscles of the floor of the mouth together with the stylohyoid and digastric muscles, the submaxillary gland, sometimes the ipsilateral half of the thyroid gland, and the parathyroid glands of that side, the fat pad of the posterior triangle of the neck, the internal jugular vein and some of its branches, the external carotid artery and some of its branches, and the deep cervical chain of lymph nodes together with their lymphatic channels.

While the addition of so extensive a procedure to the total laryngectomy may seem extremely radical, the additional amount of deformity resulting therefrom is surprisingly small. Ordinarily the procedure sacrifices the spinal accessory nerve, which results in some limitation of ability to elevate the arm, but apart from this there is relatively little disability and certainly nothing to offset the benefits of the far greater percentage of cures when the

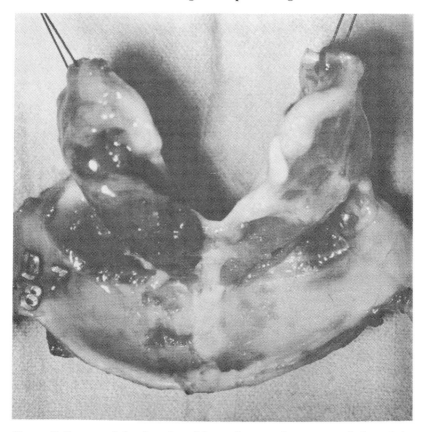

FIGURE 7. Larynx of the dog viewed from above to demonstrate fusion of the two sides. Injection of dye has been made into right side of larynx seven hours before sacrifice. The soft tissues have been separated from thyroid cartilage. In the midline the white, narrow strip of cartilage (intralaryngeal cartilage) represents the line of fusion of the two lateral halves of the larynx. The soft tissues are correspondingly joined by a fibrous raphé which is also visible.

combined operation is performed. In special cases, such as in house painters to whom normal elevation of the arm is essential, the spinal accessory nerve can be spared. Whether this significantly lessens the percentage of cures is doubtful.

Total laryngectomy requires that the end of the trachea, which is severed from the larynx at the junction of the two, be brought to the surface of the skin at the lower level of the neck, and its edges sewn to the rim of a buttonhole defect in the skin which has been prepared to receive it. This creates a breathing hole much like that of the whale. It is called a "tracheal stoma." Air passes directly through the trachea to the lungs without, of course, having passed through the upper respiratory channels of the nose, mouth, and throat.

It is this short-circuiting of the air column to an exit point below the mouth and throat which necessitates the development

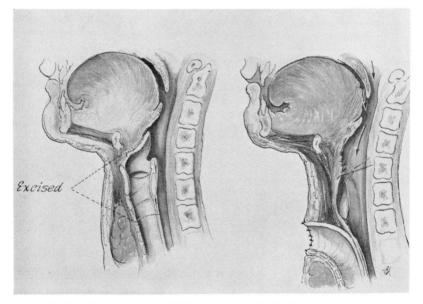

FIGURE 8. Total laryngectomy. Half section of the head and neck demonstrating the normal arrangement of the mouth, pharynx, and larynx preoperatively. On the right is the change in arrangement after removal of the larynx. The severed end of the trachea has been brought forward and sutured to a hole in the skin of the neck. The hiatus created in the pharynx by removal of the larynx is being closed with sutures.

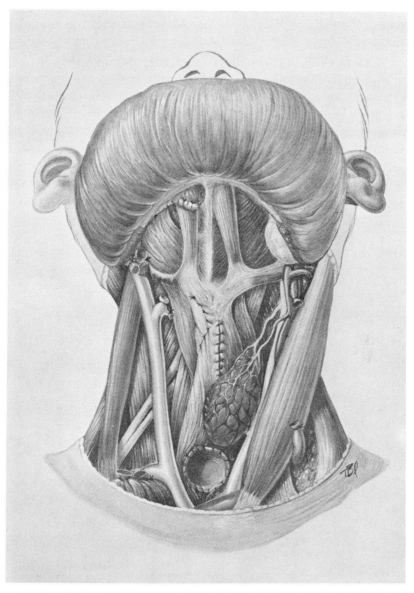

FIGURE 9. Total laryngectomy with radical neck dissection. The larynx has been removed and the radical neck dissection performed on the right side. Comparison can be made with the left side to observe the structures removed by the operation.

of esophageal speech. Air from the esophagus is forced into the mouth, vibration at the top of the gullet replacing that from the lungs.

Conley (128) attempted to overcome this difficulty by providing an independent airway from the trachea to the upper esophagus or hypopharynx. He states his purpose as follows: "It was hoped that a new operation to supply adequate air easily for phonation purposes would eliminate the gulping technique and permit the patient to talk with ease." Specifically, Conley's method consists of isolating a segment of the remaining esophageal mucosa and forming it into a mucosal tube by suturing the sides together over a mold which acts as a temporary stent. The latter

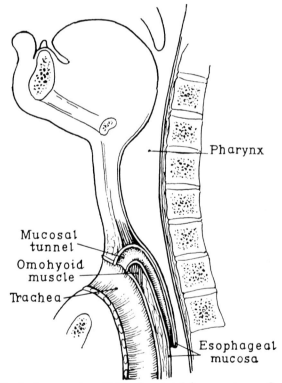

Figure 10. Conley's operation. Following total laryngectomy, Conley uses a graft formed into a tube to provide an airway between the trachea and the pharynx. The graft is either a transplanted vein or section of esophageal mucosa. Its use at this time is not intended as a routine measure.

is removed in six weeks. The free end of this tube is sutured into the posterior surface of the trachea or the skin of the neck above the tracheostoma. The fixed end opens into the pharynx. One modification of this technique utilizes one of the anterior jugular veins as a tubular graft instead of the mucosa of the pharynx. One gathers that the technique, as ingenious as it is, at this time is less than completely satisfactory and requires further development before it can be considered as effective for routine use.

Numerous other disadvantages accompany breathing through a tracheotomy fistula as compared to normal channels. The inspired air is not properly warmed, filtered, or moistened; the efficiency of the cough mechanism is markedly reduced; ability to increase intra-abdominal pressure as in childbirth or emptying the bladder and bowel is lessened and, because air does not pass through the nose, the senses of smell and taste suffer. Many people continue to smoke, but because no air can be inspired through the mouth the ability to do so is impaired. Some authors believe that the effciency of movements controlled by muscles of the pectoral girdle is diminished, but experiments by the author seem to negate this.

In addition, of course, is the obvious handicap of the need to avoid swimming and bathing in tubs which may lead to lung infections from the entrance of nonsterile water into alveoli of the lungs or even drowning. One such patient in the author's experience fell asleep in a bathtub and virtually drowned. Showers with a stoma guard are permitted.

Other complications include the invasion of the lower respiratory tract through the tracheal stoma by insects and dust. The' avoidance of this requires the use of filters such as mesh gauze held in place over the opening by tapes tied around the neck.

Following the removal of the total larynx, a hole exists in the lower pharynx representing the area closed in by the larynx itself. This is sewn together to reestablish the continuity of the swallowing passage between the oral cavity and upper esophagus. Occasionally the extent of spread of surgically treated cancer of the larynx is such that removal of portions of the pharyngeal wall or even the whole pharynx is required. Continuity of the swallowing passages, under such circumstances, cannot always be immediately reestablished. Until recently, almost all attempts to accomplish such a closure at the time of operation had failed, and patients remained with large infected openings in the neck through which saliva constantly poured. Feeding was accomplished through an indwelling stomach feeding tube, and many months passed during which skin flaps or tubes were fashioned from skin to form a new esophagus and brought from distant sites by a slow tedious process involving many surgical procedures performed at intervals.

Recently great advances have been made in this direction as well. By the use of molds and stents with overlying skin grafts, Ormerod (562), for instance, has succeeded in closing such defects rapidly and efficiently. Wookey (821) contributed a technique which re-created the swallowing passage by the use of skin tubes created from the skin of the neck. The author, following successful experiments upon laboratory animals, has contributed a method consisting of the use of segments of the largest blood vessel of the body, the aorta, preserved in the dehydrated state in vacuum tubes, to temporarily provide a continuous intact swallowing passage from the mouth to the esophagus in the chest. One end of the vessel is sewn above to the base of the tongue and the upper pharyngeal wall at the point of severance, and the lower end to the thoracic esophagus, thus bridging the gap created by loss of the lower pharynx. This is covered by the skin of the neck, and complete healing takes place permitting one to swallow normally. In the event that contraction of this vascular tube seems likely, as it often does, and satisfactory dilatation cannot be accomplished by bouginage, local skin tubes are constructed over a period of time to replace the aortic channel. Even when this is necessary, the advantages are hardly to be overestimated, primary complete healing having taken place without the presence of large infected openings in the neck. The technique, therefore, gives the surgeon an opportunity to reconstruct the swallowing passage in delayed stages while the patient swallows normally.

Subtotal Laryngectomy

As has been indicated under the historical reviews, surgeons had for many decades attempted to develop methods of surgical resection of the tumor-bearing area without sacrificing the normal channel for the passage of air. Great strides have recently been made, and many patients previously considered as requiring total laryngectomy have been spared the handicap of loss of the normal airway by less radical but more sophisticated techniques, and without lessening the cure rate. Many techniques have been proposed and used. All are designed with the same end result, that is, the creation and maintenance of a mucosal-lined, granulation-free patent channel for the passage of air between the trachea and the pharynx. The techniques utilized for this purpose are numerous, the selection depending upon the site of the lesion, its extent, and the personal preference of the surgeon.

In the simplest procedure performed for the removal of small tumors limited to the margin of a vocal cord, the thyroid cartilage is split in the midline and access thus gained to the interior. The tumor-bearing area is removed and the larynx closed. This operation of laryngofissure or thyrotomy presents no particular postoperative problem because the normal lumen and rigid walls of the larynx are not disturbed. Occasionally granulations or proud flesh repeatedly forming over the site of the resected cord are bothersome and may require removal through the direct laryngoscopy; but, ultimately, mucous membrane grows over the raw surface and healing takes place.

Sometimes if the tumor has necessitated resection beyond the midline, a small web is likely to form from one side to the other, occupying the space between the severed ends of the vocal cord. This can be prevented or later corrected by the method of McNaught, described in personal communication, which leaves a keel of metal or plastic between the cords until healing has taken place.

In any event, a fibrous band forms to replace the resected segment of vocal cord and, since the intrinsic muscles — particularly those controlling abduction and adduction through rotation of the arytenoid cartilages — have been left intact, the movements of the vocal cords postoperatively are essentially normal and the voice very good indeed. Some residual loss of quality commonly occurs so that the singing voice might be impaired and the speaking voice prove to be less pleasing. But for all practical purposes of everyday life, the degree of disability is surprisingly small.

Occasionally when the postoperative formation of proud flesh over the area of removal is excessive, healing may be long delayed. To obviate this, St. Clair Thompson (771) introduced the technique of removing that portion of the exposed cartilage underlying the resected area. This resulted in the interior of the operative site being covered by the external perichondrium rapidly, whereas its growth over the surface of cartilage is exceedingly slow. This modification, therefore, results in much more rapid healing than would otherwise be the case.

Until recently the procedure commonly used for unilateral tumors of such distribution as to be too extensive for laryngo-fissure but not sufficiently widespread to require total laryngectomy, was the removal of the involved lateral half of the larynx, not, however, including the cricoid cartilage. This was the so-called operation of hemilaryngectomy introduced by Billroth in 1878. Like all subtotal resections, its success, insofar as cure was concerned, depends upon the proper selection of cases, and since the technique makes no provision for exploration of the nodes of the neck or extension beyond the larynx, a great many failures are to be expected. Because of the unilateral distribution of the lymphatics and submucosal compartmentation of the larynx as described in previous paragraphs, this procedure will cure any case of cancer in which the tumor is actually limited to one side and has not spread beyond the confines of the larynx. The uncertainty in any given case, however, is whether or not extension beyond these limits has occurred. The operative technique ordinarily fails to establish this fact, even at the time of surgery.

From the technical standpoint, the operation of hemilaryngectomy is easily performed; but, in the author's experience, the raw surface left remaining over so wide an area results in long-delayed healing with infected granulations and only too often an inadequate airway. The voice is usable but seldom useful for professional purposes such as lecturing. This has been more or less the general experience, and the operation has for many years been in disfavor. Attempts to make up for its shortcomings by using skin grafts placed *in situ* over tampons have, to some extent, eliminated the problem of postoperative granulations and contributed to the expectation of a better airway, but the excised half of the newly formed larynx lacks rigidity and, therefore, the number of patients who can be decannulated, insofar as the tracheotomy is concerned, is limited.

Max Som (715), after removing half the interior of the larynx together with the thyroid cartilage, utilizes elements of the mucosa of the residual area for primary closure and thereby prevents the formation of granulations proportionately reducing the element of risk insofar as postoperative stenosis is concerned.

Many newer types of subtotal resections have been described by various contributors to the surgical literature. Most of these have followed the general pattern of fitting the technique to the individual case, removing that portion of the larynx deemed necessary and saving fractions of it not likely to be involved. From these salvaged segments, new pseudolarynges have been created which in some instances are adequate both for speech via normal channels and respiration without a permanent tracheotomy. In those others in which the functional result permits the normal route for speech but provides a lumen too small for normal breathing, a better, less aspirate voice is apt to result. In patients so operated upon, the normal movements of the vocal cords are ordinarily lost and the laryngeal orifice becomes a channel more or less rigid and fixed in size, the area of which needs to do for both functions. Sometimes, however, under certain conditions if one or both arytenoid cartilages have been salvaged, some degree of abduction and adduction of the fibrous bands that form to replace the vocal cord takes place. Under these circumstances, a much closer approximation to the normal physiology results, so that the size of the lumen narrows for phonation and widens for respiration. This, of course, results in a better voice and adequate respiration without the use of a tracheotomy tube. As a general rule, however, it can be assumed that after any subtotal laryngectomy, the better the voice, the less adequate the airway will prove to be.

As contrasted with the total laryngectomy which is relatively

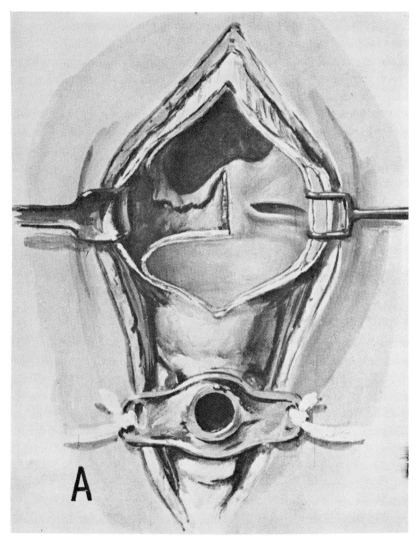

FIGURE 11. Max Som's partial laryngectomy. Front view. Cut edge of the mucosa above is sutured to the mucosa below in an attempt to eliminate raw surfaces.

simple to do, most subtotal operations require a high degree of technical skill and a detailed knowledge of the intimate structure of the larynx. The end result in patient welfare, however, is immeasurable since the loss of one's larynx is a tragedy obviously to be avoided whenever possible.

Any subtotal laryngectomy should ideally fulfill five requirements:

1. The tumor-bearing area and an adequate uninvolved margin surrounding it should be removed.
2. An opportunity must be provided at the time of surgery for an adequate examination of the remainder of the larynx and the corresponding lymph drainage areas of the neck.
3. It should provide an airway that is well-lined, rigid, and adequate not only for sound production but for respiration through normal channels as well.
4. The "glottic valve" mechanism should be preserved so that the patient retains the ability to increase intrathoracic pressure for coughing, lifting, and bowel function.
5. The ability to swallow *without aspiration* should be preserved.

Of the many techniques that have been suggested, only a few accomplish this. Hautand's (313) method literally takes the larynx apart, permitting visualization of ordinarily hidden areas in which extensions of the tumor may have grown and yet not be recognized; it permits removal of subglottic areas as far interiorly as the lower border of the cricoid cartilage, and removal of sections of that structure when required. It retains a segment of the thyroid cartilage adequate for support postoperatively and, in properly selected cases, even with widespread involvement, provides ample opportunity for complete removal of the tumor-bearing area and an adequate segment of surrounding normal tissue.

The "extended fronto-lateral partial laryngectomy" procedure described by Alonso and by Jackson and Norris (365) accomplishes essentially the same thing, but in order to encourage rapid healing and provide a lining, these surgeons use a skin graft over a stent mold after the method of Figure 13. It allows for removal of extended portions of the larynx, as determined to be necessary at the time of surgery, which is an obvious advantage. Norris reported upon sixteen such cases with only one known recurrence and a five-year follow-up cure rate of 83 per cent. This is very good indeed, particularly in that many of the cases were of extensive involvement.

In 1951, one of the present authors (JJP) (601) introduced a subtotal laryngectomy with repair and reconstruction of the laryngeal airway by a technique described under the term "laryngoplasty." This technically complicated procedure was subsequently modified in 1963 by the other author (BJB) (23). It provides for the five requirements of subtotal laryngectomy as listed previously. By the use of this technique, one can remove any part of the larynx which is determined to be involved during the operation. By reason of the elevation of broad skin flap overlying the front of the neck, all the lymphatics are exposed to direct view and palpation and, because the larynx is literally disassembled, no portion of its interior remains hidden from view. Rigidity and support are provided by maintaining the attachment of the thyroid cartilage posteriorly, then placing a bipedicled sternohyoid muscle flap inside the thyroid cartilage to fill the defect left by the removal of the tumor. The procedure provides for relining the air passage with perichondrium from the external surface of the thyroid cartilage. Mucous membrane rapidly grows over the surface of this tissue. Several steps in this operation are shown in Figure 14.

Formerly, it was felt that subtotal laryngectomy procedures must be limited to small unilateral carcinomas. However, we have been able to resect very large tumors involving both sides of the

---

————————→

FIGURE 12. Hautand's laryngectomy. From Ombrédanne, M.: *Traitement du Cancer Endolarynge*. Paris, Masson & Cie, 1930. (*upper*) This operation literally takes the entire larynx apart and permits inspection of hidden recesses into which cancer may have extended. It permits removal of tumors from the lower level of the cricoid cartilage to the upper level of the thyroid cartilage. (*lower*) A view from above showing the outline of the area resected by Hautand's technique.

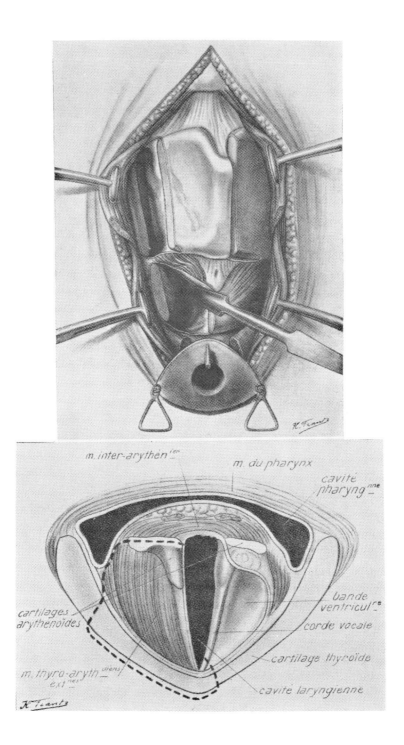

m. inter-arythèn.ien

m. du pharynx

cavité pharyng.nne

cartilages arythénoïdes

bande ventricul.re

corde vocale

cartilage thyroïde

m. thyro-aryth.iens ext.nes

cavité laryngienne

PARTIAL   LARYNGECTOMY

EXTENDED   FRONTO-LATERAL

(g r a f t - m o l d)

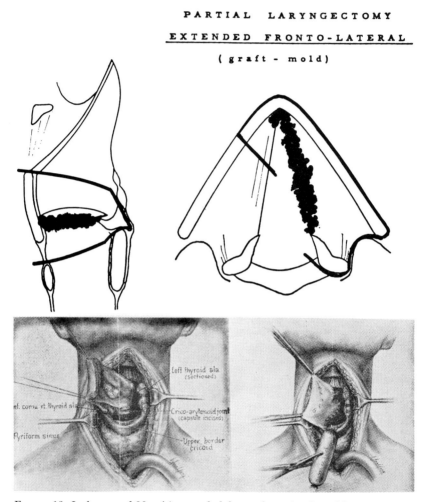

FIGURE 13. Jackson and Norris' extended fronto-lateral subtotal laryngectomy. (*upper left*) View from the side and from above demonstrating the portion of the larynx excised. This consists of the ala of the thyroid cartilage and the entire interior of the larynx on the involved side including the true vocal cord, ventricle, false vocal cord and the intrinsic muscles as well as the arytenoid cartilages. (*upper right*) Segment of the lining and thyroid cartilage is resected as far as necessary to clear the lesion. (*lower left*) Demonstration of the area to be excised freed and about to be removed. (*lower right*) Skin graft in place about to be sutured to the opposite side over a mold.

larynx which left only the posterior half of one vocal cord and one arytenoid cartilage at the glottic level. These patients have had very adequate voices and respiratory exchange with their reconstructed larynges.

Special types of partial subtotal laryngectomies serve specific purposes. One needs to be reminded that the lymphatic flow in the larynx is always from inferior to superior levels. This gives an opportunity to resect upper segments of the larynx by transverse resections either unilaterally or bilaterally. Ogura (552) has introduced such a technique removing all the larynx above the level of the true vocal cords. This removes most of the protective sphincter mechanism of the larynx, but Ogura states that after a time patients are able to swallow without the complication of food entering the airway. It is also possible to combine this type of subtotal laryngetcomy with removal of the appropriate lymphatic drainage (radical neck dissection).

In carcinomas of the epiglottis, Som (715) has performed transverse resections at higher levels to include the epiglottis; this seems to be an effective method of dealing with localized lesions of that region.

It should be stressed that modern surgical concepts no longer consider the larynx as an organ to be resected *in toto* simply because one section of it is the site of cancer. The larynx is composed of many component parts, a number of which can be spared when resecting a tumor-bearing area. These segments can be utilized to reconstruct a suitable airway always adequate for speech, and often for both speech and respiration through normal channels. On the other hand, when it is established that the distribution of the lesion is such that total laryngectomy needs to be performed, it is often well to remove the corresponding lymph drainage area as well so that a radical neck dissection, sometimes bilateral, is often considered an essential part of the operation. The concept has served to improve the surgical results so that the overall cure rate of laryngectomy is now 60 to 70 per cent and, in less extensive cases, one can hope for a cure rate exceeding 90 per cent.

Like carcinoma everywhere, early recognition is the key to success. The longer carcinoma remains unrecognized and untreated, the more radical the surgery will need to be, and greater the likelihood of failure. One needs to bear in mind that the usual site of origin of cancer of the larynx is in the anterior segments of the true vocal cords, and because of the overhanging of the epiglottis, this region is the most difficult to see with a laryngeal mirror. Fortunately, cancer originating here gives early warning by producing changes in the voice. Therefore, unexplained hoarseness in which the anterior commissure of the larynx cannot be adequately visualized by mirror examination indicates further examination by tomographic x-rays and direct laryngoscopy.

$\longrightarrow$

FIGURE 14. The authors' subtotal laryngectomy with laryngoplasty. This operation is performed through a very cosmetically satisfactory "collar incision" which permits examination and palpation of the lymphatic structures of both sides of the neck. The thyroid cartilage is split in the midline, preserving the external perichondrium of the thyroid cartilage for use as a new lining. Resection of the interior of the larynx as required is accomplished, and then the laryngeal interior is reconstructed using a bipedicled sternohyoid muscle flap to fill the surgical defect and the thyroid ala to provide support and rigidity.

A. Palpation for enlarged nodes along the jugular vein.

B. Elevation of external perichondrium of the cartilage.

C. Incision of thyrohyoid membrane for direct inspection of the tumor. The internal perichondrium is then elevated from the thyroid cartilage on the side of the lesion.

D. Resection of the true cord, ventricle, and lower half of the false cord but preserving the overlying thyroid cartilage.

E. Incision to create a bipedicled sternohyoid muscle flap with perichondrium on its deep surface.

F. An elevator is passed through the sternohyoid muscle incision to facilitate placing the bipedicled muscle flap inside the denuded thyroid ala.

G. Muscle positioned within larynx, and mucosa is carefully sutured to perichondrium.

H. After a stent has been placed in the larynx, the thyroid alae are reapproximated.

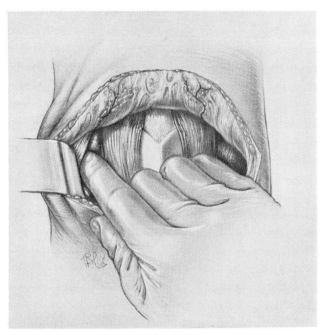

FIGURE 14A.

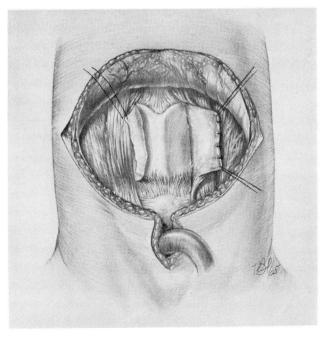

FIGURE 14B.

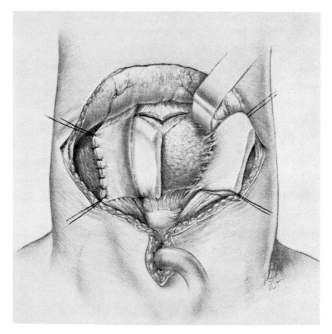

FIGURE 14C.

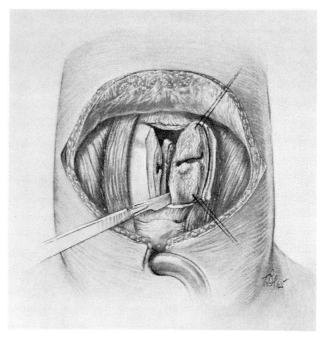

FIGURE 14D.

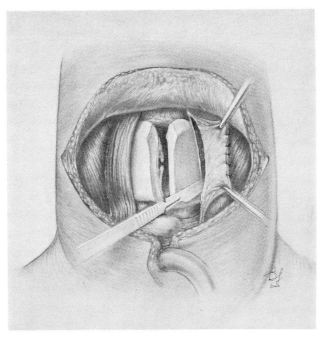

FIGURE 14E.

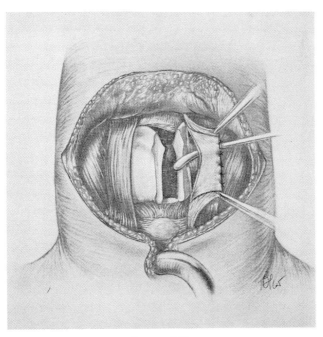

FIGURE 14F.

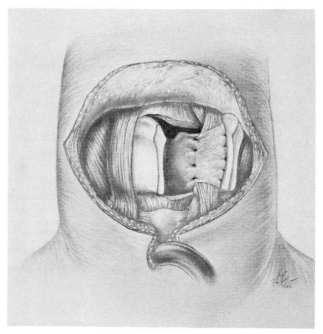

FIGURE 14G.

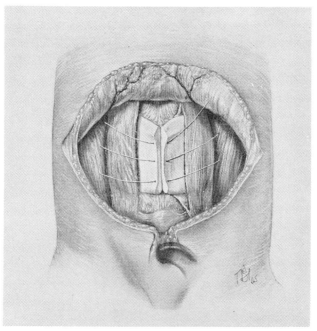

FIGURE 14H.

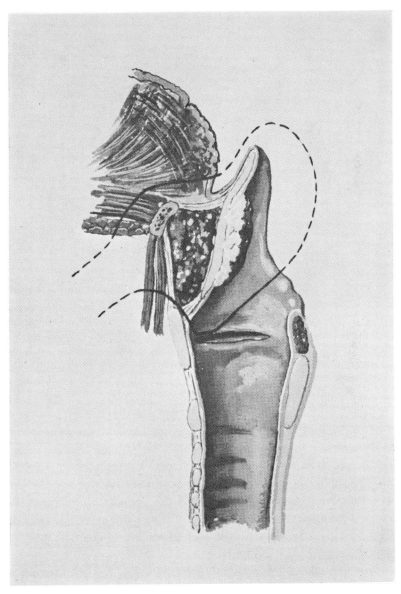

FIGURE 15. Lateral view of Som's total epiglottectomy for cancer of the epiglottis.

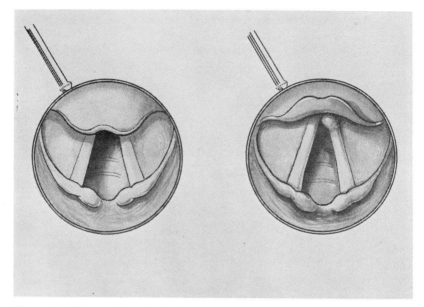

Figure 16. Mirror view of the larynx. On the left is demonstrated a mirror view of the larynx with the epiglottis overhanging the anterior commissure which is the usual site of early cancer of the vocal card. On the right is demonstrated the view of the cancer hidden by the overhanging epiglottis. It is essential for proper diagnosis that the entire length of the vocal cord be visualized.

Summary

In the matter of cancer of the larynx, surgical research is constantly striving to perfect operations which permit more nearly normal speech than is possible with total laryngectomy. Such advances must be made upon the basis of greater knowledge of tissue space, lymphatic flow, the biology of the tumors, and other basic factors. The greater our knowledge of these, the more likely is the surgeon to achieve his ultimate goal of obtaining the best possible voice without undue jeopardy to life.

The first recorded subtotal laryngectomy was performed in 1833. The subsequent history of the procedure is given in some detail. Subtotal resections permit phonation through normal channels even though the airway might not be adequate for normal respiration. The need of esophageal speech is thereby eliminated.

The advantages are therefore obvious, provided the recurrence rate is not thereby increased.

Any subtotal laryngectomy should provide the surgeon with an opportunity to observe and palpate the lymph nodes of the neck, whereas other very large ones may not do so for long periods of time.

Recently gained knowledge concerning the anatomy of spread of cancer within the larynx and its route of escape beyond has resulted from experiments upon the larynges of dogs, pigs, human cadavers, and the living human subject. These experiments have demonstrated that: (1) the interior is divided into a number of submucosal compartments which are more or less isolated from one another insofar as communication between them is concerned; (2) the lymphatic flow within the boundaries of the larynx is from inferior to superior; (3) there is no communication between the deep lymphatics of one side of the larynx and the other, but the surface lymphatics through the mucous membrane do communicate freely across the midline. This isolation of one half of the larynx from the other results from the embryonic development of each side separately. Fusion takes place by an intermediary embryonic "intralaryngeal cartilage," to which each side fuses separately.

The disadvantages of breathing through a tracheotomy fistula are cited. These require that every effort be made to reestablish the continuity of the larynx to such a degree that an adequate airway will be provided. There is then described a type of subtotal laryngectomy designed by the authors which has accomplished this in the vast majority of cases. Other similar operations enjoying equal success have been described by other authors and are cited.

In conclusion, it is stressed that the larynx is to be considered as composed of a number of parts, many of which can be preserved and reformed into a new pseudolarynx. The concept that it is a single organ requiring removal *in toto* simply because one section of it is the site of cancer is an outmoded concept that needs to be discarded.

Chapter III

First Experiences with the Asai Technique for Vocal Rehabilitation after Total Laryngectomy

ALDEN H. MILLER

L ATE IN 1965, it was my privilege and pleasure to see and hear a sound movie by Dr. Ryozo Asai, in which he demonstrated a method of providing laryngectomized patients with an almost normal voice. The basis of his technique was the construction of a dermal tube from the upper end of the trachea into the hypopharynx. When the lower tracheal fistula, which had been placed for breathing, was closed with the patient's finger, air could then be expired up the dermal tube and into the pharyngeal cavity with sound produced there and transformed into speech. The voices of these patients had an excellent quality and a wide range of pitch. They could sing, whistle with ease, and speak sentences of average length with normal pauses for inspiration.

In January of 1966, I used Dr. Asai's technique for the first time, performing the first stage at the conclusion of a wide-field laryngectomy. The final stage in nine such patients has been completed, and the first or second stage in another ten patients has been done. The first six have excellent voices, far superior, in my opinion, to the average esophageal voice after laryngectomy. There are two slight inconveniences for these patients. First, one has to use a hand to close the tracheal opening when he talks and, second, he has to press the skin manually over the upper end of the dermal tube sometimes when swallowing saliva or liquid foods.

Technique

The technique consists of three stages or operations. The first stage is employed at the end of an ordinary wide-field laryngectomy. After removal of the larynx, the open end of the trachea is sutured to the skin opening of the midline of the neck in the

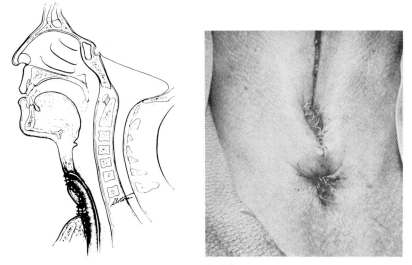

FIGURE 17. End of first stage.

usual fashion. When using the usual midline vertical skin incision for the laryngectomy, the open end of the trachea is placed a centimeter or two higher than usual. This necessitates some closure of the lower end of the incision below the tracheal stoma thus being formed. A permanent tracheal stoma is then made through the fourth or fifth tracheal ring with 2 cm of skin between it and the upper opening. This will be the patient's permanent opening for breathing during the remainder of his life. The stoma made above it will become the lower opening of the final dermal tube into the pharynx. This completes the first stage of the technique.

The second stage consists in making, a month or so later, a fistula into the pharynx, suturing mucosal edges to skin edges. This fistula should enter the pharynx just under the overhang of the bulge posteriorly of the base of the tongue or the remaining shelf of floor of valleculae.

The third and final stage, another month or so later, forms a tube of skin with its lower opening being the upper tracheal stoma and its upper opening being the fistula into the pharynx. This tube is formed by making a vertical skin incision 1 cm on

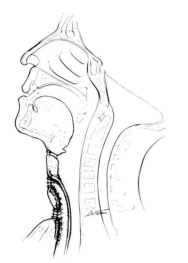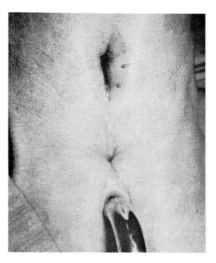

FIGURE 18. End of second stage.

each side of the midline of the neck and curving these incisions around and above the pharyngeal stoma by 1 cm, and below and around the upper tracheal stoma by the same centimeter. The cut edges of this island of skin are then approximated and sutured vertically in the midline. Thus is formed a tube of skin connecting the uppermost end of the trachea and the pharynx. The remaining cut skin edges are now closed vertically in the mid-line over the dermal tube, burying it.

The first patients have taught us certain rules and measurements to follow during the surgery of each stage and in postoperative management. In the first stage, it is preferred to insure that the lowermost opening, the permanent tracheal stoma, be a little smaller than usual. A diameter of about 12 mm is probably best. This may mean the use of a number seven or eight laryngectomy tube instead of a number nine. The middle stoma, the uppermost end of the trachea, should end up being about 6 mm in diameter. This may necessitate the wearing of a small plastic tube or plug in this opening during the month intervening between the first and second stage and even that month between the second and third stage of the technique.

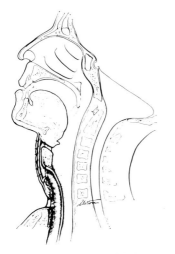

FIGURE 19A. End of third stage.

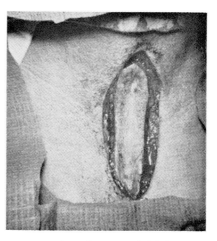

FIGURE 19B. First step of third stage.

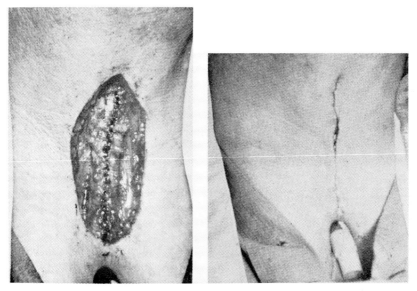

FIGURE 19C. Second step of third stage. FIGURE 19D. Third step of third stage.

In the second stage, one should attempt to place the pharyngeal stoma in such a way that it runs downhill from its skin opening to its pharyngeal opening. The pharyngeal opening should be placed just under the ledge formed by the remaining floor of the valleculae left at the conclusion of the laryngectomy. This, of course, necessitates leaving some of this anterior floor when the larynx is severed from the base of the tongue. A direct laryngoscope should be used during this second stage of surgery to direct the insertion to this spot of a large needle through the skin of the midline of the neck at just about where the skin of the neck angulates with that of the underside of the floor of the mouth. This is about the level of the removed hyoid bone. When the needle is angulated properly, an incision then follows it into the pharynx. The skin opening is kept high when mucosal edges are sutured to skin edges. This pharyngeal stoma is made vertically with a vertical diameter of 1 cm. The pharyngeal stoma will narrow in the postoperative course of this second stage. Ideally, it should end up remaining with a diameter of about 4 mm. This may necessitate the wearing of a plastic tube or plug in this stoma or in daily dilations for a few weeks.

During the third operation, the dermal tube is formed over a section of plastic tubing having an outside diameter of 6 mm. This tubing is left in place for two or three weeks from just where it can be seen through the permanent tracheal stoma, up the dermal tube, into the pharynx and standing with its upper end at the level of the top surface of the tongue. Suture is tied into both ends of it to form an endless circle in order to replace it if it moves upward or downward. At the conclusion of the third stage, the patient will immediately be able to talk in a hoarse whisper, even with the plastic tube in place.

Results

The first two patients, the two who have had their final operation completed longest, have excellent voices. They can talk with inflection and a wide range of pitch and tonal quality and can even sing. Final surgery on the oldest patient has been completed twenty nine months, and his voice continues to improve. The second patient has had her procedures completed twenty four months and she, too, has continued to have a voice that steadily improves in loudness, range, and singing ability; she has retained her southern accent. The third and fourth patients' voices were not as strong the few months following their final surgery but are steadily improving.

The first patient has no difficulty with swallowing solids but sometimes must use digital pressure over the skin over the upper end of the dermal tube with drinking some liquids. The second patients must use the digital pressure with the swallowing of all liquids. The third patient, in whom for the first time the pharyngeal stoma was deliberately slanted downward from the skin, has absolutely no leak of either liquids swallowed or of his saliva. None of the patients report any cough resulting from the trickling down of saliva and none have had any infections of the respiratory tract. All report that talking seems to keep the dermal tube clear of saliva.

The first two patients state that talking is much easier when they leave their laryngectomy tubes in place and occlude its opening rather than occluding the tracheal stoma when the tube is not in place. The first patient obtains his loudest and clearest voice when he uses a second finger for digital pressure over the lowermost end of the dermal tube in order to narrow its lumen. Interestingly, the greatest vibration of the dermal tube is felt where it is narrowed.

Only the first patient has had hair grow up through the pharyngeal stoma from the dermal tube. This has given him no symptoms, and the hairs are being evulsed at direct or indirect laryngoscopy.

Hinged trapdoor tracheotomy tubes or tubes with diaphragms have been used so as to allow the patients to close off the tube on expiration and thus talk without having to use one hand to close the opening of the tracheotomy tube. Their voices have remained almost the same as with digital closure of the stoma, but both patients report an uncomfortable suffocating-like feeling after a minute or so or talking as if they could not expire enough air. They have insisted that these hinged tubes are too uncomfortable.

It seems certain that soon a trapdoor can be fashioned that will allow the patient to flip it open to relieve this sensation.

Conversion

Can this technique be used to convert the patient who has had the usual laryngectomy with just the formation of one rather low-lying stoma? A pharyngeal fistula was placed in one such patient as a second stage. At the time of the third and final stage, the tracheal stoma was freed in its anterior 180° of circumference and the trachea was elevated 2 to $2\frac{1}{2}$ cm. A new lower permanent tracheal fistula was formed, and the upper two openings connected in forming a dermal tube in the usual manner. This patient had an uncomplicated postoperative course and has a good voice. The actual steps of this technique will be reported later. In a second such patient, the bridge of skin between the two tracheal stomas broke down.

Summary

My first experiences with the usage of the Asai technique for vocal rehabilitation of the laryngectomized patient have been recounted. I am convinced that these patients will continue to have excellent voices, far superior to those with esophageal voices. However, these patients must put up with some discomforts in order to have these voices. Instead of one, there will be three operations and convalescent periods. Patients must use one hand to close the tracheal stoma when talking, and some will experience slight annoyance in having to close the dermal tube with digital pressure when swallowing liquids. These drawbacks must be pointed out to the patient contemplating such surgery. The patients who have an excellent esophageal voice will probably not choose to be converted to the Asai technique, nor would I encourage them to have the conversion, although I think we will be able to convert almost any laryngectomized patient.

Observations of the Senior Author

During the fall of 1968, Dr. Snidecor served as a guest professor at the University of Kyoto and had an opportunity to visit the University of Kobe where he observed Dr. Asai perform the third stage of his operation. The patient phonated while still on the operating table.

A selected group of Dr. Asai's seventy patients was studied. The following points directly related to Dr. Miller's presentation can be made.

1. The majority of the subjects used digital pressure to control the swallowing of liquids.
2. Some speakers used pressure on the dermal tube to alter pitch and loudness. One especially effective speaker placed the thumb and an index finger of the right hand at the top of the dermal tube where it turns inward and downward toward the hypopharynx.
3. It appears that hair within the dermal tube is not a problem in the Japanese male. This may be due to the fact that he is, generally speaking, less hirsute than the American male.
4. The Kobe research group has developed a valve for the stoma that remains open for normal breathing and closes automatically when breath pressure is increased for speech. The valve must be carefully adjusted and requires care in cleaning. It is this writer's opinion that the valve would be a nuisance except for those rare cases in which both hands and speech would be needed concurrently.
5. Detailed voice studies, which are reported elsewhere, support the observations made by Dr. Miller.
6. Japanese observers have also noted that voice improves gradually over a period of four months or more. It is possible that a speech pathologist who is versed in alaryngeal speech techniques might speed the learning period and, in general, minimize the trial-and-error aspects of relearning.

Chapter IV

Surgery and Speech, the Pseudoglottis, and Respiration in Total Standard Laryngectomy

EVELYN ROBE FINKBEINER

Types of Surgery in Total Laryngectomy as These Relate To Learning of Esophageal Speech

ESOPHAGEAL VOICE, the substitute voice which utilizes the patient's own pseudoglottis, is generally considered far more natural and dependable than that produced with the aid of mechanical devices. Unfortunately, not all laryngectomized persons are able to develop it. Despite the amount of knowledge regarding esophageal speech which has accumulated in the last fifty years, one of the important questions which remains to be answered is why some individuals are able to learn to use the new voice without undue difficulty while others, who appear equally well motivated, fail in their efforts to acquire it. Psychological reasons for such failures have been stressed in the literature, while relatively few opinions are to be found concerning the influence which operative techniques may have.

At the time when laryngectomized patients were first learning to use esophageal voice, Stern, one of the early investigators in the field, expressed the belief that the new voice might be dependent upon the anatomic conditions created during the operation. It was not until many years later, however, that further opinions regarding this question were published. Typical of these views was that of Kallen, who felt that the surgeon should be interested in preparing the patient as favorably as possible for the phonetician: "Every fold of mucous membrane, every favorably placed cicatricial band, every muscle or muscular remnant, may serve as the basis for the development of a pseudoglottis" (380).

Recommendation has been made by a number of surgeons (248, 290, 429, 452, 479, 521) that the greatest care be taken during laryngectomy to spare the fibers of the cricopharyngeal muscle, and, if possible, to preserve the integrity of its innervation. There were also those who advocated preservation of the sternohyoid and thyrohyoid muscles, suturing them to the anterior wall of the pharynx as a later aid in relaxing the tonic closure of the cricopharyngeus and facilitating aspiration of air for speech.

The deliberate creation of a fistula during or following laryngectomy as an aid to speech development was suggested by Guttman (290) and by Jackson and Jackson (363).

Guttman was motivated by the experience of a laryngectomized patient who, because he objected to an artificial larynx, had taken a heated ice pick and passed it through the trachea to the hypopharynx several times, thus forming a permanent fistula. He was able to use the fistula to provide an air supply for an excellent substitute voice.

Guttman's procedure was to insert a needle electrode through the tracheal stoma and up behind the remnants of the epiglottis so that the opening would be partly protected from the ingress of food and water to the trachea. Within two weeks, the electrocoagulated tract usually developed a definite fistula. After formation of the fistula, the patient could be taught to block the tracheal stoma with a finger and to force the air up along the fistulous tract. Pitch could be varied to some extent by flexion of the head, thus varying the tension on the fistula.

For several years, the possibility of creating a passage which would permit air to flow through the trachea without strangulation received no further attention. In 1958, however, Dr. John Conley, of the Pack Medical Group, reported results of a new surgical technique designed to accomplish this aim. In place of a fistula, a mucosal tunnel is constructed through the wall of the cervical esophagus without the disadvantage of having food and saliva spill into the trachea or onto the neck (128).

It should be noted that all those whose opinions have been cited regarding the creation of optimal postoperative conditions for esophageal voice have stressed strongly that excision of malignant tissue must always be the primary consideration in laryngectomy, and that conservation of tissue as an aid to later voice acquisition, although desirable, is necessarily a secondary concern.

TABLE I

Subject	Sex	Age at Time of Laryngectomy	Type of Laryngectomy	Postoperative Recovery Factors Which Might Have Influenced Speech Development	Preoperative Speech Training	Postoperative Speech Training (Number of Lessons)	Present Evaluation of Speech Fluency*	Comments
1	M	27	Laryngectomy and right radical neck dissection			17 class	c	
2	M	48	Wide field			4 individual	g	
3	F	32	Laryngectomy and left radical neck dissection			2 individual 1 class	g	Prefers to use electrolarynx because of gastric discomfort accompanying esophageal voice production.
4	M	51	Modified narrow field			6 individual	d	
5	M	39	Narrow field			8 individual	g	
6	M	48	Modified narrow field			4 class	g	
7	M	57	Modified narrow field			3 individual 1 class	g	
8	M	56	Wide field			16 individual	f	
9	M	48	Narrow field			2 individual	g	
10	M	71	Modified narrow field	Some swallowing difficulty		3 individual 10 class	f	Has hearing loss.
11	M	60	Partial laryngectomy (Epiglottis and cricoid remain)	Infection about cricoid cartilage		5 individual	d	
12	M	60	Narrow field			9 individual	f	

Case	Sex	Age	Field	Notes		Treatment	Code	Remarks
13	F	52	Wide field and thyroidectomy			8 individual	g	
14	M	47	Narrow field			16 individual	f	
15	M	53	Narrow field			1 individual	g	
16	M	54	Narrow field			9 individual	f	
17	M	51	Wide field	Fistula		10 individual	g	
18	M	51	Narrow field			5 class	c	
19	M	54	Narrow field			8 individual	g	
20	M	60	Wide field			3 class	f	
21	M	49	Narrow field			2 individual	g	
22	M	68	Wide field		1 individual	5 individual	g	
23	M	57	Narrow field	Fistula postponed speech training		2 individual / 7 class	e	
24	M	48	Narrow field			8 individual	g	
25	M	59	Wide field			9 individual	g	
26	M	56	Narrow field			1 individual / 8 class	g	
27	M	58	Narrow field			4 individual	g	
28	M	70	Narrow field	Fistula		2 individual / 6 class	g	
29	M	53	Narrow field			1 individual / 7 class	g	
30	M	64	Wide field			4 individual	a	Became discouraged. Will not continue lessons.
31	F	29	Modified wide field			5 individual / 2 class	f	
32	M	70	Modified wide field			5 individual / 2 class	b	

*See Table V in the present chapter.

The effect which combined laryngectomy and radical neck dissection might have upon later development of a substitute voice should also be considered. Unfortunately, very little information on this aspect of the subject is available. An effort to gather such data was made in 1952 by Robe, Moore, Holinger, and Andrews (622). In their study, thirty-two persons who had been laryngectomized within the preceding five-year period were selected as subjects. Data concerning the type of laryngectomy, postoperative recovery factors, and preoperative speech training were obtained from the case histories and operative reports provided by the surgeons who performed the laryngectomies, while information regarding the amount of postoperative speech training which the subject had received was obtained from their teachers.

The information from the several sources was classified under the headings as shown in Table I. Only significant characteristics of the group and simple relationships between type of laryngectomy were considered.

It is of interest to examine the sex ratio and age range represented: twenty-nine of the group were male and three were female. The preponderance of males bore out the findings of other investigators who have reported sex ratios incident to cancer of the larynx varying from 9:1 to 14:1 (364). Review of the ages of the subjects at the time of laryngectomy revealed a range of

TABLE II

INCIDENCE OF LARYNGECTOMY RELATED TO AGE IN
EXPERIMENTAL GROUP

20-30	*30-40*	*40-50*	*50-60*	*60-70*	*70-80*
27	32	47	51	60	70
29	39	48	51	60	70
		48	51	60	71
		48	52	64	
		48	53	68	
		49	53		
			54		
			54		
			56		
			56		
			57		
			57		
			58		
			59		
2	2	6	14	5	3

twenty-seven to seventy-one years, with the majority in the fifty- to sixty-year group (Table II). A recent tabulation by Harrington (309) indicates a 9:1 sex difference throughout the age range. Most important, he found with a group of 306 patients, sampled without regard to ability to pay, sex, age, color, and so forth, that exactly one-half of these patients fell above and below the age of sixty. J. Perelló (583) of Barcelona found comparable statistics for a sample of 213 laryngectomees studied at the San Pablo Hospital, Barcelona. His median case is also at the sixty-year level. In 1950, Gardner reported that 70 per cent of laryngectomees studied by him fell below the age of sixty. It appears that Gardner's and Robe's average ages would be revised upward if more general public clinical cases were added to the samples. Recent publicity has been given to Paul Streble (445) who was operated on at six years of age for cancer of the larynx and who shortly became a highly skilled speaker.

Classification of the group according to type of laryngectomy is shown in Table III. Postoperative complications, such as infection or fistula, occurred in five patients but had no adverse effect in at least three who developed excellent speech.

The speech of each subject was observed in a variety of speaking situations, and his fluency evaluated in terms of the scale (shown in Table V). Speech fluency ratings ranged from the lowest on the scale (no sounds produced), to the highest (fluent, nonhesitant speech). Eighteen of the thirty-two received the highest rating as shown in Table V. The number of speech lessons which the person had had (Table IV) did not seem to be related to speech fluency; some were fluent after one lesson, while others needed more instruction.

With regard to the relation of the type of laryngectomy, the following observations were made on the ability of the subjects to

TABLE III
INCIDENCE OF TYPE OF LARYNGECTOMY IN
EXPERIMENTAL GROUP

Laryngectomy and Radical Neck	*Wide Field*	*Narrow Field*	*Modified Narrow Field*	*Partial Laryngectomy*
2	8	17	4	1

TABLE IV
CLASSIFICATION OF AMOUNT OF GROUP AND INDIVIDUAL
POSTLARYNGECTOMY SPEECH INSTRUCTION

| | Class | Individual | Individual and Class | |
			Individual	*Class*
	3	1	2	1
	4	2	3	1
	5	2	3	10
	17	4	2	7
		4	1	8
		4	2	6
		5	1	7
		5	5	2
		6	5	2
		8		
		8		
		8		
		8		
		9		
		9		
		9		
		10		
		16		
		16		
Total number of subjects	4	19	9	
Average number of lessons	9	7	8*	

*Individual and group combined.

TABLE V

CLASSIFICATION OF SUBJECTS ACCORDING TO
SPEECH FLUENCY

a. No sounds produced	1
b. Partial control; single sounds under fair control	1
c. Simple words produced	2
d. Combines 2-3 words	2
e. Some sentences used	1
f. Sentences consistently used	7
g. Fluent, nonhesitant speech	18

develop speech: Seventeen of the subjects had had a narrow-field laryngectomy, in which the thyrohyoid and sternothyroid muscles are usually preserved. The fact that ten of the seventeen received the highest rating on the fluency scale, and that three others were given the second highest rating, suggests that a relationship between the type of laryngectomy and the later ability to develop substitute voice may have existed in this group. That substitute voice does not always depend on the presence of the strap muscles, however, is evident from the number of those who developed fluent speech following wide-field laryngectomy, and from the fact that one of the two who had had laryngectomy with radical neck dissection was able to develop fluent speech.

The majority of the subjects available for the study had a narrow-field operation. This did not reflect conservatism in surgery but is probably due to the fact that, for the most part, they were referred as private patients whose lesions generally received earlier attention than might have been true of a similar group selected from a large charity service.

Mention should be made of the five subjects who had experienced a modified narrow-field laryngectomy. The modification in both types consists essentially of resection of the middle section of the hyoid bone and tapering of the pharynx downward. It is possible that this type of surgery should provide a positive aid to postoperative speech development when the pseudoglottis is formed at the pharyngo-esophageal (P-E) junction. For this reason, it is regrettable that more patients who had undergone this type of surgery were not available for the study. The fact that three of the group experienced difficulty in learning to use a substitute voice, largely because of the infirmities of age such as hearing loss, makes it impossible to evaluate the direct effect of the operation on later speech. The remaining three of the group who were free of such problems developed fluent speech after fewer than the average number of lessons.

It was not always possible to ascertain from the operative reports the exact percentage of the cricopharyngeus that was preserved; nor is it possible to estimate the amount of actual functioning muscle which is present after the healing process has been completed. No conclusions can be drawn, therefore, in regard to the role it may have played in the postoperative speech development of the group. Seeman (666), in a recent report on 342 cases, supports the results of this survey. He reports: "The various methods of operation themselves have no influence upon the functional results of esophageal speech. After all, the site of the operation lies above the mouth of the esophagus. It is only necessary to

preserve the cricopharyngeal muscle and not to destroy its innervation provided by the recurrent nerve."

Precethel, a surgeon and colleague of Professor Seeman, has
worked to develop a technique of laryngectomy specifically aimed
toward later voice development. One purpose of his method is to
avoid the siphon-shaped deformity that very often appears at the
level of the superior esophageal sphincter following healing after
the operation and which negatively influences the development
and quality of esophageal voice. His is a functional reconstruction
of the hypopharynx. By preservation and careful suturing of the
laryngeal muscles, he makes the anterior wall of the hypopharynx
firmer and forms a pseudoglottis of chosen shape and tension between the preserved part of the lamina of the cricoid and the
upper esophageal sphincter the insertions of which he sutures to
the capsule of the thyroid gland. Precethel (599) is of the opinion
that the pseudoglottis thus created permits the optimum vibratory
conditions, thus resulting in good voice production.

Vrticka and Svoboda (792), also members of the Phoniatric
Research Institute of Charles University in Prague, have reported
on the postlaryngectomy speech results of a group of seventy men
(34 to 74 years of age with an average age of 56.5). Gluck's wide-
field laryngectomy had been performed in most cases, while Precethel's functional reconstructive laryngectomy had been performed in nine of the patients. A thorough otolaryngologic, phoniatric, and x-ray examination was made of all patients. The quality
of speech was evaluated according to the classification of speech
fluency given earlier in Table V.

Of the seventy patients examined, fifty-three (75.71%) attained esophageal speech sufficient for current conversation (f and
g in Table V), and eight patients (11.43%) attained speech sufficient for basic communication (d and e). In four patients
(5.71%), the speech was insufficient for practical communication
(a, b, and c), and in five patients (7.14%) who did not appear for
further controls the results of rehabilitation could not be evaluated.

In summing up the results of the study, we may say that the
types of surgery did not in themselves appear to determine the

relative excellence of the speech result nor the amount of speech training necessary to achieve satisfactory postlaryngectomy speech.

Site of the Pseudoglottis

Interest in discovering the site or source of vibration in substitute voice production has led to speculation and study from the time that laryngectomized individuals first learned to use such voices. Location of the pseudoglottis is, of course, important to the surgeon, who believes that every effort should be made to preserve the structure involved, as well as to the teacher of postlaryngectomy speech. It has been difficult to reach general agreement on a specific site, however, because of the unique difficulties involved which often lead to inconclusive results. When mirror examination of the lower pharynx is attempted, for example, movements of gagging and the presence of secretions often obscure the vibrating structures. Protrusion of the tongue for viewing the hypopharynx ordinarily modifies or eliminates posterior glossal vibration, although in some cases inspection of the area during sound production is possible without tongue protrusion.

Various anatomic structures which may serve as a pseudoglottis have been reported and include the following sites: (1) between the base of the tongue and the posterior wall of the pharynx, (2) between the back of the tongue and the tightly stretched velum, (3) between strongly contracted portions of the inferior constrictor, (4) between the epiglottis and the two folds formed laterally from the musculature of the pharynx, (5) the esophageal mouth of Killian, between the folds of the cricopharyngeus. Sometimes there is no real glottis in some, rather the sound of eructated air (522). Kallen adds that "every fold of mucous membrane, every favorably placed cicatricial band, every muscle or muscular remnant, may serve as the basis for the development of a pseudoglottis" (380).

The most generally held opinion is that the cricopharyngeus is the usual site of the pseudoglottis. Seeman made one of the first scientific studies of the problem and concluded that the anatomic and physiologic conditions of the esophagus meet the requirements for the production of substitute voice in every respect. This was because of its capacity to (1) hold more than a few cubic centimeters of air; (2) be filled with air quickly and voluntarily; (3) expel air under control; and (4) set the pseudoglottis into vibration by providing the necessary air current, thus fulfilling the requirement that the air chamber be caudal to the pseudoglottis (325).

The majority of those who regard the cricopharyngeus as the most frequent site of the pseudoglottis base their conclusions, at least in part, on roentgenological observations which, despite many limitations, have provided the most objective evidence thus far.

Damsté (151) compared radiographs of eight good speakers with those of eight poor speakers and noted that "The shape of the pseudoglottis is fully determined by the cricopharyngeus muscle. The prominence formed by this muscle is, in most cases, before the fifth and sixth cervical vertebrae, in poor speakers, often lower." With regard to the group of poor speakers, he observed that an important characteristic was the formation of a bulge in the ventral side of the pseudoglottis in which secretions easily accumulate, giving the voice a bubbly-mucous sound.

In 1952, the author of this chapter, together with Moore, Holinger, and Andrews, used roentgenography to study the pseudoglottis in sixteen laryngectomized speakers (622). Five films were made of each subject. Film 1 was taken with the subject at rest prior to air intake for speech. Film 2 showed the structures just after the subject had taken in a maximum amount of air in preparation for phonation. Film 3 was exposed during production of the vowel *ah*. Film 4 followed immediately after the production of the vowel.

The subject's position was changed for the fifth film so that he stood at a 45° angle to the chest table. This provided a full-length view of the esophagus. He was given the same instructions as for film 2, and the exposure was made when he had taken in the amount of air preparatory to phonation.

The following observations were made from the series of films obtained: (1) The films of the good speakers showed a constriction of the pharyngo-esophageal air column at the approximate

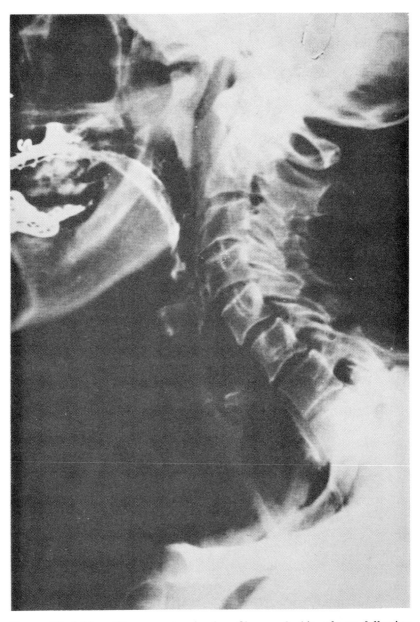

FIGURE 20. Subject XI, a superior speaker, film no. 2. Air column following maximum oral intake of air preparatory to sound production.

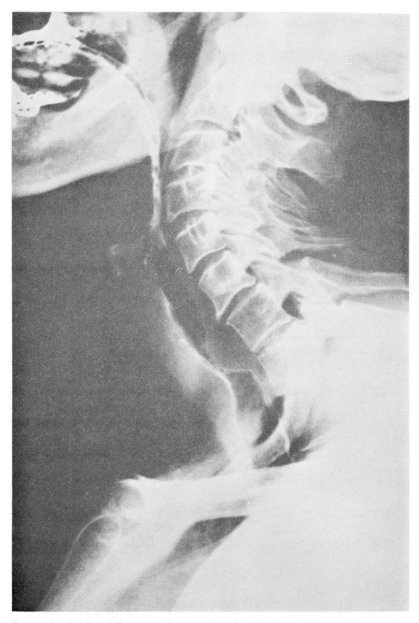

Figure 21. Subject XI, a superior speaker, film 3. Constriction of the esophageal air column during production of vowel sound *ah*.

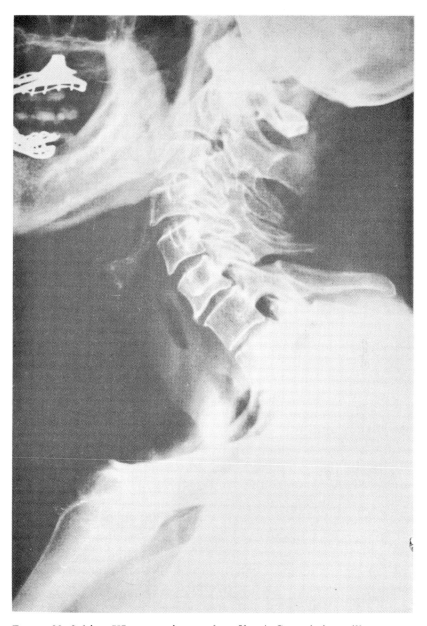

FIGURE 22. Subject XI, a superior speaker, film 4. Constriction still apparent following phonation; air column below decreased in size.

level of the fifth vertebra and the cricopharyngeal muscle. (2) The films of the good speakers also showed an air column of adequate size below the pseudoglottis. Figures 20 and 21 illustrate the presence of a visible air column in subject XI, a speaker with an excellent esophageal voice of more than adequate volume. The formation of this column of air below the pseudoglottis appears to be analogous to the use of subglottal air in normal phonation. Such a column was absent in the films of the poor speakers. The x-rays of subject XV, a poor speaker, are shown in Figures 23, 24, and 25. This speaker had inconsistent control of sound production, and his voice was often too weak to be heard. It appears therefore that an adequate sized air column is important in the production of a good esophageal voice.

The larger, oblique films, made at the point of maximum intake of air for speech, showed that air is generally visible throughout the length of the esophagus rather than in the upper part alone.

The roentgenographic studies just discussed were dependent on single radiographs. These yielded much valuable information for analysis but were inadequate in that they showed limited aspects of the function of the pseudoglottis. Radiocinematography, therefore, which has become available in recent years, provides an admirable means of studying the pseudoglottis in action.

One of the most outstanding of such films is that of van den Berg, Moolenaar-Bijl, and Damsté made in 1955 — a cine x-ray with synchronous sound of the region of the pharynx, the pseudoglottis, and the esophagus. Others who have used the new method are Di Carlo, Amster, and Herrer (171); Diedrich and Youngstrom (172) in the United States; Schlosshauer and Möchel (644) in Germany; and Hodson and Oswald (325) in England.

In their film, Hodson and Oswald observed that during speech the sphincter at the upper end of the esophagus was in a constant state of activity, varying rapidly in tightness with the modulations of speech. They also noted that, although the length of the various sphincters varied only slightly from case to case, the position of the center of the lumen differed considerably. A possible explanation offered for the different varieties of sphincters is that actual struc-

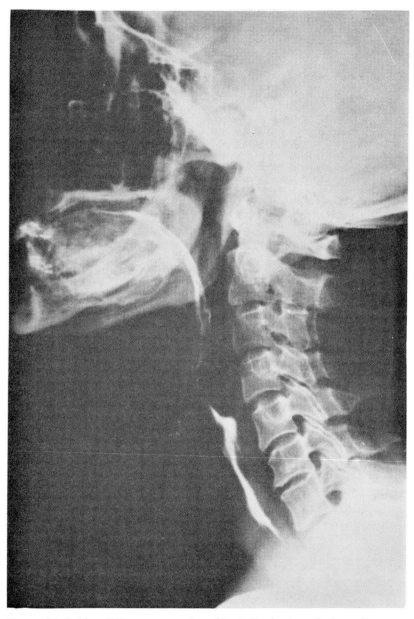

FIGURE 23. Subject XV, a poor speaker, film 1. Beginning of phonation, note absence of air column in cervical esophagus.

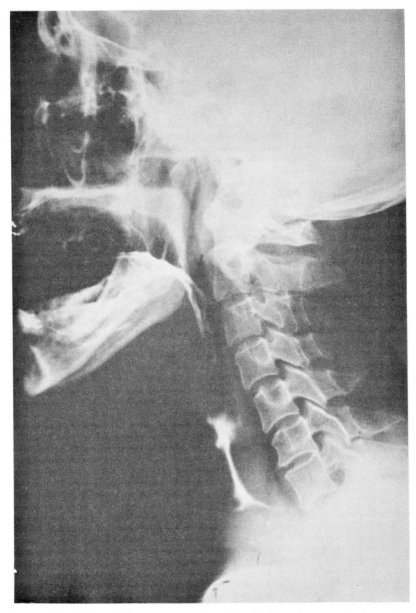

FIGURE 24. Subject XV, a poor speaker, film 2. Second stage of phonation, tongue is raised, the pharynx narrowed.

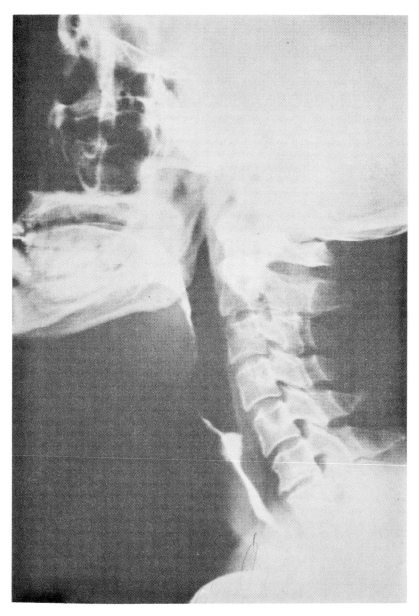

FIGURE 25. Subject XV, a poor speaker, film 3. Mouth open, pharynx constricted, esophageal column compressed from below.

tural changes may have been brought about during the operation. In one instance the esophagus remained intact along its wall, while in others local scarring was noted, causing an irregular contraction.

While fluoroscopic and roentgenological studies have provided the most objective data thus far, there is still room for research employing other techniques. Motion picture photography is one.

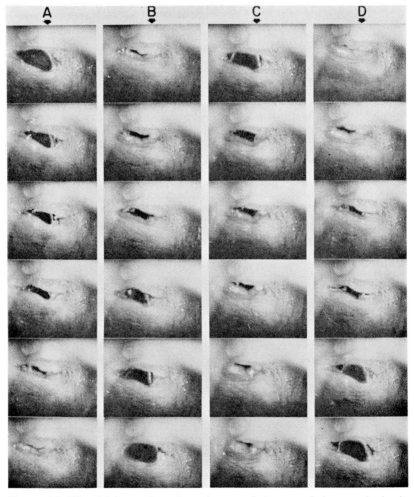

FIGURE 26. Ultra high-speed motion pictures of the top of the pseudoglottis. Note bubbles of mucus present at the top of the pseudoglottic column. *Courtesy of Henry J. Rubin, M.D.*

In their 1952 study, Robe *et al.* applied the same procedures used for laryngeal photography to obtain visual evidence of the functioning pseudoglottis. Eight subjects who had sufficient practice in tolerating the laryngeal mirror while producing sound were instructed to sustain the vowel *eh* while the camera was in operation. Magnetic tape recordings of the sound produced were made concurrently with the films.

In the analysis of the films, the pattern of movement most often observed was that of a circular drawing together of the walls of the pharynx, and a marked bubbling of saliva as the sound was produced, followed by a drawing apart of the pharyngeal walls. The nature of movement and the presence of mucus are shown especially clearly in a recent ultra high-speed film, by Rubin (633), reproduced in Figure 26.

The eight individuals who participated in this procedure were excellent speakers. Their films indicated that in every case, with the possible exception of one, the movement just described took place at the level of the cricopharyngeus.

Diedrich and Youngstrom (174) in 1966 noted that the P-E junction is most often at the level of the fifth and sixth cervical vertebrae. It is noted from their data that if the cervical levels from 4 to 7 are grouped, the P-E junction will fall therein over 90 per cent of the time. They also note that the junction will be influenced by the nature of the vowel, by swallowing, blowing or the modified Valsalva maneuver. Bork, in an unpublished study, appears to be in agreement when she notes that there are marked differences in the morphology of the speaking mechanism from speaker to speaker as well as from phonation to phonation.

Coordination of Speech with Respiration

Loss of the vocal function as a result of laryngectomy involves not only removal of the sound-producing mechanism, but also, in general, exclusion of the continued use of the trachea and the lungs to supply air for audible speech. Except in the case of the laryngectomized speaker who employs the reed type of artificial larynx, or who has had the modified surgery performed by Dr. Conley, the process of pulmonary respiration is separate from that of phonic respiration.

This changed relationship between breathing and speaking frequently presents discouraging difficulties to the individual who is learning to use a substitute voice. It also provides one of the greatest points of controversy with regard to theory and methods of teaching postlaryngectomy speech, that is, whether air is inspired through the tracheostoma to the lungs at the same time that air is drawn orally into the vicarious air chamber, and whether air is expired from the lungs as the oral air is used in speaking.

From 1930 to the present time, there has been great interest in the development of programs for teaching postlaryngectomy speech. Nearly all such programs have included recommendations concerning breathing and speech coordinations.

Kallen, in 1934, as part of his proposed program, recommended the reconditioning of phonic respiration as the patient's first task, even though it meant dissociating "the behavior patterns of a lifetime." The dissociation was necessary, he thought, because the old respiration habits would hinder production of the new voice and cause fatigue. Alternative methods to achieve the reconditioning were suggested: either the patient could be taught to hold the thorax in the position which follows inspiration and, while holding this position, to take in air for speech; or the patient could take in air for speech after the lungs had been emptied of breath. He added that the latter method might be easier, but in either case it was necessary to continue to practice until conscious control of the process had been achieved (380).

Jackson and Jackson (363), in their program for teaching a patient to develop articulate speech without a larynx, gave the following instructions:

> The patient should be taught to inhale air into his esophagus by the expansion of his thorax in the ordinary breathing way, but at the moment of inspiration, the cannula must be obstructed with the finger. The air not being permitted to enter through the trachea will enter through the mouth or nose and be drawn into the esophagus.

The method is based on the theory that when air is first inspirated, then swallowed, inspiration and deglutition are not synchronized through being made to occur consecutively. One of the chief advantages of the method is that "it forestalls the acquisition of the undesirable habit of air intake between short words or between syllables of longer words" (363) .

Koepp-Baker (401) advised the speech clinician to make a direct attack upon the patient's "tendency to breathe through the tracheostomy tube during the esophageal voice production. This results in air turbulency at the orifice of the tube and obscures much of his speech." The physiological basis for such advice he explained as follows:

> In normal speech, controlled expiration is an unconscious process. The cerebral cortex integrates the total synergy of respiration, valvulation at the larynx, and the chewing, sucking movements in the mouth for normal speech production. When the total speech pattern is modified by loss of the larynx, and the esophagus and pharynx are used for phonation, this totality must be fractionated and respiration must be inhibited.

Holding the breath while belching air is described by Gardner (238) as one of the most important techniques for laryngectomized speakers to learn. The reason for its importance is that it permits the speaker "to use the abdominal wall and chest muscles to exert pressure with the greatest efficiency. If air is breathed out while trying to belch, the decreasing volume of the chest cavity tends to lessen the tension and pressure for belching."

Stetson, one of the chief proponents of synchrony between pulmonary and phonic respiration, employed apparatus specifically designed to make an objective and qualitative analysis of postlaryngectomy speech. The three forms he studied were (1) the buccal whisper, (2) voice produced with an artificial larynx, and (3) esophageal voice.

With reference to esophageal speech, he found the chest action for each syllable and the breathing movements for phrasing comparable to those of normal speech, although movements of the sternum and epigastrium appeared to be somewhat more vigorous. This may explain why students of esophageal voice at first tire easily, become dizzy, or have other transient symptoms.

Stetson's (730) spirometric records showed that only a little air is taken into the esophagus (from 2-5 cc) . He observed that "this intake is made frequently and rapidly with the mouth and velum closed; it often fuses with the movement of the consonant. Intake of air every few syllables is the one thing contrary to ordinary speech which the patient has to learn."

With regard to volume of air taken into the esophagus and the number of syllables which can be produced, Howie (336) observed that a speaker can usually produce three or four syllables on one intake of air and probably uses 1 cc of air for each syllable.

It is interesting to compare the foregoing figures with those given in a report of more recent work by Snidecor and Curry (708). In their study of a group of six superior esophageal speakers using a sensitive electropneumograph and phonophotographic equipment, the lowest average value was found to be 3.8 syllables; the highest, 8.7 syllables, with the speakers averaging 4.98 words per air-charge. Snidecor, in Chapter V, specifically points out dangers in overgeneralizing on information from a very select group. No mention of synchrony or dyssynchrony of pulmonary and phonic respiration is made by the authors in their original study. Further analysis of their pneumographic information, however, indicates that the two types of respiration were synchronous.

Another proponent of synchrony is a Dutch investigator, Moolenaar-Bijl (515). In the course of her investigations, she found that phonation always appeared to be coupled with expiration. Two types could be distinguished according to whether the swallowing or sucking technique was used. When spirometrical curves were made of the speech of the patient who used the swallowing method, it was found that the mouth of the esophagus closed after phonation, which coincided with expiration, and remained closed until the next swallow which occurred synchronously with inspiration. Observation of the esophageal curve when the patient was not speaking revealed absence of movement. This was confirmed by x-rays which showed no air in the esophagus while the patient was silent.

Analysis of spirometrical curves of the speech of a patient who used the sucking technique led Moolenaar-Bijl to conclude that a parallelism exists between the tracheal and esophageal movements. In speech as well as in quiet respiration, the curves of the trachea and the esophagus traveled up and down together. When x-ray photographs were made of this patient, the esophagus was observed to be filled with air before and during speech. In the process of speaking, air was pushed out of the esophagus with pulsatile movements of the tongue or lips, which were sometimes identical with the articulation of initial plosives.

Among others who have used spirometry to obtain evidence concerning the relationship between phonic and pulmonary respiration in esophageal speech are Anderson, Di Carlo, Amster and Herrer, and Robe.

Anderson (10) employed pneumopolygraphs to make simultaneous records of the mouth, thorax, and abdomen. His recordings showed intake of air into the mouth to be neither significantly synchronous nor dyssynchronous with inspiratory movements of the abdomen and thorax. In general, the abdomen and thorax exhibited synchrony of gross patterns, but not when the tracings were compared for small detail.

Di Carlo, Amster, and Herrer (171) in 1954 reported that their spirometrical curves provided evidence of synchrony between pulmonary and phonic respiration.

Robe *et al.,* in their 1952 study, employed a graphic recording apparatus and motion picture photography to analyze the process. Twenty-three laryngectomized persons who were classified as fair, good, or superior speakers were selected as subjects for both parts of the study.

The first procedure involved the modification of equipment ordinarily used for studying the normal respiratory function. The second respiration records were of particular interest because they resulted from the use of equipment and procedures different from those employed previously (see Fig. 27). For the most part, investigators have had to depend on pneumographs which fastened about the chest and abdominal areas.

The recording of the speech and respiratory data for each subject for the first procedure consisted of four sections. During section I, the subject was asked to breathe quietly without speaking. For section II, he was asked to count from one to five at his usual rate and volume. In section III, he repeated five words from a standard "phonetically balanced" list, while in section IV, he repeated each of eight, five-syllable phrases equated as to time and intensity. All sounds produced by the subject were recorded on magnetic tape.

In analyzing the completed records, the volume of air taken in during the inspiration phase of each cycle of pulmonary respiration was measured in cubic centimeters for each of the four sec-

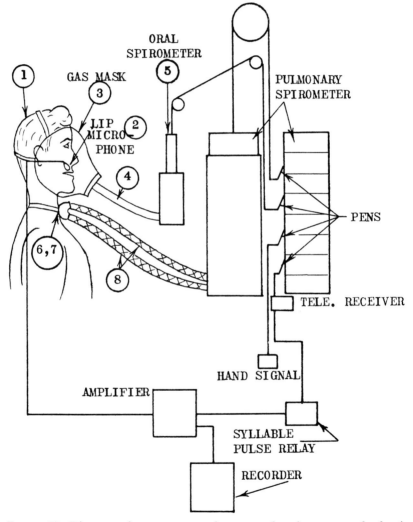

FIGURE 27. Diagram of apparatus used to record pulmonary and phonic respiration.

tions. The volume of air taken into the mouth for speech and the volume of air used in each speech unit were also measured in cubic centimeters. Finally, careful study and comparisons of the oral and pulmonary curves were made to determine how many occurred synchronously and how many did not.

According to the results of the respiratory tracings, pulmonary and phonic respiration occur together. The tracings also showed a wide variation in the volume of pulmonary and oral air, with no relation between amount of air taken into the lungs and that drawn in through the mouth for speech. Furthermore, the fluency of a speaker seemed independent from the volume of air drawn into either the lungs or mouth.

The second procedure used in the study involved motion picture photography and speech recordings. As in the first precedure, twenty-three subjects participated. Each subject was prepared in the following way: (1) The tracheostoma and the area around it were uncovered so as to be clearly visible. (2) A square of single-thickness facial tissue slightly larger than the tracheostoma was secured along its top edge with Scotch® tape, which was then attached to the neck just above the tracheostoma in such a way that the tissue would be moved readily by the respiratory air. (3) The subject was then asked to read the same words and sentences which had been used in the first procedure, followed by two short paragraphs. A film and sound recording were made as each subject read (Fig. 28).

The films, which were analyzed frame by frame, together with the sound recordings, showed a drawing inward of the tissue curtain as the speaker took in air both orally and through the tracheostoma in preparation for the following word or phrase. The curtain moved outward and remained so as long as the subject was speaking, that is, pulmonary air was being expired through the tracheostoma at the same time that the phonic air was being expired through the mouth.

The results of this study add another bit of evidence in favor of synchrony between oral and pulmonary respiration. There is much to be said, however, in favor of not taking too definite a stand in the controversy of synchrony versus dyssynchrony. Exam-

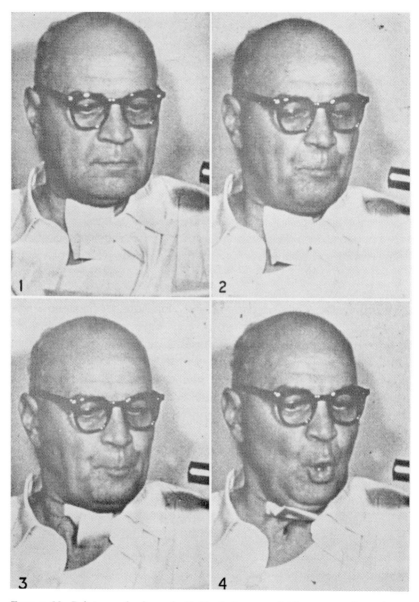

FIGURE 28. Prints made from individual frames of 16 mm moving picture film giving visual evidence of relation between phonic and pulmonary respiration. 1. Quiet breathing. 2. Intake of air. 3. Start of phonation with raising of flap. 4. Phonation with flap blown out.

ples of both undoubtedly exist, and it is highly probable that some speakers shift from one to the other. Clinical experience teaches us how helpful the dissociation may be in certain cases where efforts to conform to the old breathing habits result in excessive air noise at the tracheostoma. It is very possible that some of those who have recommended that the laryngectomized speaker learn to dissociate the two processes would not advocate that the dissociation be continued after the new speech is well established.

Chapter V

Time and Rate in Superior Esophageal Speech

John C. Snidecor

I N 1956, THE AVAILABLE materials related to esophageal speech had little to offer in the way of direct information on time and pitch, and it was necessary to set up research projects to answer important questions regarding these aspects of speech. The findings herein reported have been published in less detailed form and with less discussion in references 708 and 709. The experimental procedure, as well as selection of subjects, is discussed in some detail with the hope that others will complete comparable studies on average or adequate speakers, and with female speakers.

In 1964, Isshiki and Snidecor (356) reported in detail on speakers who ranged from adequate to superior (see Chapter IX). However, the only known study specifically on female speakers is that by Gardner (232), in which he is concerned with social and psychological problems rather than with speech in the descriptive sense.

It cannot be overemphasized that we were searching for facts about the *superior esophageal speaker*. It was felt that defining high-level performances would establish the boundaries for skilled performances and serve as goals for those in the process of learning to speak. Many esophageal speakers get along very well indeed without achieving the level of performance herein described.

The critical questions which we sought to answer were, How many words and syllables can be spoken per charge of air? How long does it take to charge air? What rate in words per minute can be achieved relative to normal speech? What characteristics of pitch level and variability can be anticipated in esophageal speech (see Chapter VI) ?

Six superior esophageal speakers read speech samples of adequate length for which norms for rate (159), breathing (707), and pitch (200) were available for normal and superior speakers.

Selection of Subjects

An initial group of fifty-two satisfactory performers from southern California was obtained through contact with otolaryngologists, speech therapists, the Veterans Administration, the American Cancer Society, the Lost Chord Club of Los Angeles, and the New Voice Club of San Diego. This group was screened successively to twenty-three and, finally, to ten performers. At this stage the following passage from Fairbanks (200) was recorded for each of the ten performers:

> When the sunlight strikes raindrops in the air, they act like a prism and form a rainbow. The rainbow is a division of white light into many beautiful colors. These take the shape of a long round arch, with its path high above, and its two ends apparently beyond the horizon.

These ten recordings were presented, when necessary, by mail, to eight skilled and experienced judges, and included the following directions:

> Please number your papers from one to ten.
> You will presently hear ten brief readings of esophageal speech. These recordings have already been screened for general effectiveness from 23 performances which in turn were screened from 52 performances. This indicates that all of the final samples are reasonably effective for the type of speech under consideration.
> Please rate each speaker for general effectiveness on a one to five rating scale. One equals good, two equals fair, three equals average, four equals good, and five equals excellent. Judge on these samples only, not on other samples of speech that you have heard.
> A brief word about general effectiveness. Its first attribute is intelligibility, but consideration is also given to those attributes of rate, loudness, pitch, quality, and articulation that make the contest easy to assimilate without stress or discomfort on the part of the speaker.
> Do *not* penalize for misreading or mispronunciation.
> You will hear all performances through once before being asked to judge. Record your judgments only on the second playing of the record.

On the basis of these judgments, six speakers were selected and utilized for the data reported in Chapter VI.

All of the speakers were males with at least four years of experience with esophageal speech. Three of the speakers were experienced teachers of esophageal speech. There were excellent female speakers in the original group, but none appeared to match the performance of the male subjects. Six judges were requested to differentiate female voices from the male voices on the basis of recordings alone. Their complete lack of success tends to indicate marked similarity in the voices of male and female esophageal speakers. This tentative statement is very much subject to check through further experimentation, although it is supported by West (810) and others who have perceived no pitch difference between male and female voices.

Each of the six speakers performed at the highest level of esophageal speech as defined by Wepman, MacGahan, Richard, and Shelton (807). In other words, they spoke with continuity and without consciousness of the act of swallowing and eructation. The speech was easily and naturally produced, without apparent thought or effort.

The six speakers were "inhalers" or "swallowers." At the time the records were made (1956), none were aware of the plosive charging method, nor did they appear to use this method. As of 1968, the author is convinced in retrospect that the speakers used a combination of methods.

Experimental Procedure

The air-charges were recorded by means of a sensitive lightweight electropneumograph placed high on the chest and similar in design and construction to that previously described by Snidecor (707) for the recording of the breathing cycle for superior speakers. In this present study, an intensity modulated 1,000 cycle tone served as an air-charge signal and was recorded on one channel of a dual channel magnetic tape recorded while speech was being recorded on the other channel. At a later time the information on each channel was transferred to the moving photographic tape or a Miller Light Writer traveling at 45 mm per second which supplied a visual record of air-charging and speech that was amenable to measurements. The rise in esophageal air pressure which actuated the pneumograph is described by Bateman, Dornhorst, and Leathhart (42) as "always accompanied by a sharp expiratory effort and loss of air from the lungs." This puff of air was audible and served to check the electrical recording. The recording of this puff might serve as an economical and reasonably accurate index of air-charge where it appeared desirable to make time estimates based on larger samples of speech. It was assumed, of course, that pulmonary air and esophageal air were synchronous in their outgoing phase. This assumption will not hold for all levels and varieties of speakers.

While recording both his voice and air-charges, each speaker performed "as if speaking to an audience of twenty-five people." First, the subjects were requested to count to ten as many times as possible on one air-charge. The best of three trials was selected for study. Counting is commonly practiced and demonstrated by esophageal speakers. It will be noted that the count to ten required the speaking of eleven syllables. Second, each subject read and was recorded for the "Rainbow Passage" (200), attempting to air-charge at points he had marked as representing his best spots to pause for air. This performance can be dismissed briefly, but not thoughtlessly, by noting that these skilled speakers did not predict with any degree of success when they were going to take an air-charge. Those learning esophageal speech frequently mark passages and take air accordingly. Their skilled counterparts are no more conscious of air intake than normal conversational speakers. Third, each subject read the "Rate Passage" (200) with a break for rest at the end of the first paragraph. All temporal data, except counting, are based on the results from this passage, a sample of which is presented later in this chapter.

Measurements were made directly from the photographic record with a simple analogue computer that read directly in seconds and decimals thereof. These results were checked against a one-tenth-of-a-second time line recorded on the photographic tape.

Experimental Results

One of the best general measures of efficiency in speech is rate. Darley (159) established norms for the passage in question for normal speakers and found that the zero percentile was represented by 129 words per minute, the fiftieth percentile by 166 words per minute, and the one hundredth percentile by 222 words per minute. Franke (217), in an investigation of the judgment of rate, found that critical listeners judged rate too rapid if it exceeded 185 words per minute or too slow if it was less than 140 words per minute.

Perusal of Table I, item 1, indicates that these superior esophageal speakers ranged from 85 words per minute to 129 words per minute for an extended performance. For the brief, fifty-six-word "Rainbow Passage," speaking rate was somewhat more rapid than for the long passage. The range was from 108 to 137 words per minute with a median rate of 122.5. No speaker exceeded Darley's fifth percentile, nor did any speaker achieve a rate that would have been judged adequately rapid in terms of Franke's data. Some 120 words per minute, or 2 words per second, is the rate at which efficient secretaries take shorthand. This rate is not slow enough to disturb the average listener. In 1965, Snidecor and

TABLE I
TEMPORAL RELATIONSHIPS

Speaker Number	*1*	*2*	*3*	*4*	*5*	*6*	*Superior "Normal" Speaker*
1. Words per minute	120	114	85	109	120	129	140 to 185
2. Count, best of three trials	10	8	10	4	10	7	40 (estimate)
3. Mean words per air-charge	4.2	5.2	2.8	2.9	6.3	3.5	12.5
4. Range in words per air-charge	1–10	1–10	1–5	1–5	3–15	1–8	2–36
5. Sigma, words per air-charge	1.8	1.9	1.0	1.0	3.0	1.4	4.9
6. Mean syllables per air-charge	5.8	7.6	3.9	3.8	8.7	5.2	17.5 (estimate)
7. Range in syllables per air-charge	3–12	2–13	2–6	1–7	4–22	2–11	2–50 (estimate)
8. Sigma, syllables per air-charge	2.11	2.57	1.13	1.21	4.05	1.95	No data
9. Mean pause time for air-charge	.54	.76	.63	.42	.80	.64	.75 to .94
10. Mean duration of air-charge	1.54	1.75	1.04	1.00	2.25	1.25	4.19
11. Mean pause time for phrases	.72	1.13	1.05	.62	1.06	.76	.63

Isshiki (711) studied a superior male speaker who read a long passage at the rate of 153 words per minute, which placed him well within the range for rate of normal speakers. This was of course a remarkable performance, but it can be duplicated by a number of superior speakers when short phrases are considered such as, "How are you?" "I'll see you Wednesday" "Goodbye till then." Too much should not be made of rate: speaker three (Table I) was consistently judged as superior to speakers four, five, and six; yet his rate of 85 words per minute was considerably lower than the rates 109 words per minute, 120 words per minute, and 129 words per minute for these other speakers.

The question obviously arises, Can the esophageal speaker speed up his rate? The answer is that he can do so only within narrow limits without sacrifice of loudness or suitable phrasing. This fact was borne out by trial runs for more rapid rate which were largely unsuccessful. This lack of modifiability is readily explained by the need for frequent air-charges on the part of even highly efficient esophageal speakers.

Item 2 in Table I, that of counting, gives some idea of this problem as will further information in Table I. None of the six speakers exceeded the count of ten (11 syllables) in the three trials allowed each speaker. Speaker five insisted that he could count to at least thirty without an air-charge. The electropneumograph proved that small air-charges were taken after the count of ten. This speaker was completely unconscious of this fact until he saw evidence of the air-charges on the instrument following the experimental run. It will be noted, however, that speaker five did read as high as twenty-two syllables on one air-charge (a figure exactly equal to the count of ten repeated twice, which contains 22 syllables due to the 2 syllables in the digit seven).

These and following data must be interpreted in relationship to the experimental situation lest the results be challenged by those who insist that advanced esophageal speakers produce two hundred syllables with one mouthful of air, and that they can count to seventy on one air-charge. The esophageal speakers in this study were held to a loudness level suitable for an audience of twenty-five people. A check of sound level pressures indicated that they maintained these levels. Lowered intensity might well increase somewhat the number of syllables spoken. As has been stated, these superior speakers, without exception, took small charges of air efficiently and unconsciously. The superior speaker using normal breath while reading the same passage did not begin to produce the syllables per breath claimed for some esophageal speakers.

Table I, item 3, indicates that mean words per air-charge range from 2.8 to 6.3 for esophageal speakers with 12.5 mean words per breath for normal breathing superior speakers. The extreme range for one esophageal speaker was 15 words (22 syllables), whereas one exceptional superior speaker under identical conditions spoke 36 words (50 syllables). These differences can be shown graphically by comparing the two passages below from Fairbank's *Voice and Articulation Drill Book.* The oblique lines in the first passage represent the air-charges taken by an efficient esophageal speaker who charges as frequently as most of his selected colleagues. The lines in the second passage represent the breaths taken by a superior, normal breathing speaker who breathes as frequently as his selected colleagues.

> Your rate of speech will be adequate / if it is slow enough to provide / for clearness and comprehension, / and rapid enough to sustain interest. / Your rate is faulty if it is too rapid / to accomplish these ends. / The easiest way to begin work / on the adjustment of your speech / to an ideal rate / is to measure your present rate / in words per minute / in a fixed situation / which you can keep constant over a number of trials. / The best method / is to pick a page / of simple, factual prose / to be read. / Read this page in your natural manner, / timing yourself in seconds. / Count the number of words on the page, / divide by the number of seconds, / and multiply this result by sixty / to calculate the number of words per minute. / As you attempt to increase / or retard your rate, / repeat this procedure / from time to time, / using the same reading material, / to enable you to check your success. /

> Your rate of speech will be adequate if it is slow enough to provide for clearness and comprehension, / and rapid enough to sustain interest. / Your rate is faulty if it is too rapid to accomplish these ends. / The easiest way to begin work on the adjustment of your speech to an ideal rate / is to measure your present rate in words per minute in a fixed situation which you can keep constant over a number of trials. /

The best method is to pick a page of simple, factual prose to be read. / Read this page in your natural manner, timing yourself in seconds. / Count the number of words on the page, divide by the number of seconds, and multiply this result by sixty to calculate the number of words per minute. / As you attempt to increase or retard your rate, / repeat this procedure from time to time, / using the same reading material, to enable you to check your success. /

Performance one for the esophageal speaker demanded thirty charges of air, whereas performance two for the normal speaker demanded only eleven breaths, yielding word-breath scores of four and twelve for the 159-word passage.

Here it must be emphasized that the typical and adequate esophageal speaker will pause for far more air-charges than did the superior performer. If an esophageal speaker were to double (or slightly more than double) the number of air-charges to sixty or seventy-five, he could still speak in an adequate manner.

Figure 29 illustrates the performance of each group of speakers in regard to the range and mean values of words per air-charge. The normal speaker reads aloud with an average of 12.54 words per breath, but has a wide range of performance, and tends to utilize breathing phrases of seven and fourteen words. The superior esophageal speaker averages 4.98 words per air-charge and has a much narrower range of performance.

Further information in Table I on syllabic performance is presented as description in addition to the grosser but more commonly used measure of words. Our syllabic values, item 6 of the table, are somewhat higher than those found by Stetson (731) who stated a limitation of from three to four syllables, whereas our lowest average value is 3.8 syllables, and our highest 8.7 syllables per air-charge. The number of speakers is greater in this study, and also the speech sample is much larger. The data of Bateman, Dornhorst, and Leathhart (42), based on three subjects and short speech samples, agree with our data insofar as these are comparable. Our information, even when extreme values are considered, is far more conservative than some information given recent wide publicity. For the average speaker we are inclined to believe that Stetson's values are quite adequate.

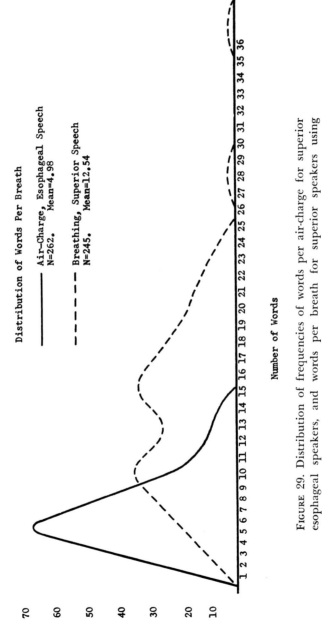

FIGURE 29. Distribution of frequencies of words per air-charge for superior esophageal speakers, and words per breath for superior speakers using normal breathing.

Esophageal speech despite frequent air-charges can be relatively efficient and pleasant to hear. How can this be true? Table I, item 9, answers this question in part. The skilled esophageal speakers gulped air in from .42 to .80 seconds, mean values considered. Damsté (150), at Groningen, reports comparable values and high speed air-charges at approximately .17 second. This is rapid air-charging — fully as rapid in fact as most normal speakers breathe for speech, although it must be added that superior, normal speakers usually breathe only at phrasal limits.

If an esophageal speaker speaks at the rate of 120 words per minute, and stops for air after each five words, he would stop twenty-four times for one-half second or a total pause time for air of only 12 seconds in one minute. Actually, he does not perform in such a consistent manner, for like the normal speaker he pauses for emphasis as well as breath at the ends of phrases which are defined for our purposes in this study as occurring at punctuation marks. Several studies indicate that the normal speaker is phonating or voicing about 70 per cent of his speaking time. The superior esophageal speaker cannot come up to this standard but will not fall far below it.

As indicated in Table I, item 11, these phrase-limiting pauses are markedly longer than the pauses for air-charging alone, in fact, approximately 1.41 times as long, ranging from one average of .62 to an average of 1.13. No exactly comparable figures can be stated for normal speakers, but pauses for phrases judged as such 50 per cent or more of the time average .63 second; whereas pauses infrequently judged as limiting phrases averaged only one-tenth of this value (706). In brief, both classes of speakers pause appropriately for phrases, but it appears that the superior esophageal speaker pauses longer than the normal speaker in order that such pauses can contrast with pauses that are for air-charges only.

The value of .63 seconds for phrasal pauses for the normal speakers is shorter than the average time utilized for breathing, which is probably explained by the fact that the normal speaker pauses for a number of phrases without taking a breath at these pauses.

As indicated in item 10, the superior esophageal speaker can utilize his air-charge for approximately one and one-half seconds (1.00 to 2.25) during which time he averages from 2.8 to 6.3 words. This contrasts with the normal speakers who utilize their breath for 4.19 seconds and speak 12.5 words. If relative time or words per air-charge is taken as a measure of efficiency, the normal speaker is from two and one-half to three times more efficient than the esophageal speaker.

It is probably much more reasonable to use total words per minute as a measure of efficiency and compare the average for esophageal speech of 113 words per minute with the rate of 166 words per minute for the average normal speaker. When this is done, the normal speaker speaks at only 1.47 times the rate of the esophageal speaker, or conversely the esophageal speaker is 80 per cent as fast as the average normal speaker. The fact that the esophageal speaker will often be judged as too slow (200) is of little consequence if his efficiency is relatively satisfactory, and it appears to be quite satisfactory for speech samples of three hundred words. It is obvious that any speech sample of over three hundred words would apply only in some type of public-speaking situation.

Most skilled esophageal speakers are fatigued at the end of a three hundred-word passage if they have been required to maintain a relatively high loudness level.

Summary and Discussion

1. The subjects in this study spoke relatively easily and were no more conscious of the "breathing" function than normal speakers. This lack of awareness in taking an air-charge is the result of much practice and long experience. It well may be that this is the most important criterion of having become a successful speaker.

2. Three speakers counted to four, seven, and eight respectively, and three speakers counted to ten on one air-charge. It should be emphasized that many esophageal speakers insist that they can make much higher counts. We doubt that the count of approximately twenty to twenty-two can be exceeded without at least an unconscious air-charge.

3. The speakers averaged five words (4.98) per air-charge,

and performances averaged about 120 words per minute. In terms of syllables, an average and realistic figure for superior speakers would not exceed 6.5 syllables per air-charge.

We did not have detailed information on average esophageal speakers, but we do know from observation that the level of performance here reported is unnecessary for satisfactory speech. For example, one of the highly rated speakers spoke at only 85 words per minute. However, his high rating was likely due to very clear articulation. There is no magic in a long phrase. Clearness, ease of speech, and reasonable rate in words per minute should take precedence over any struggle to break records in regard to words per air-charge.

4. The air-charge was taken in about one-half second, a more rapid performance than that of the normal speaker inhaling for an intraphrasal breath pause. Damsté in particular supports this finding. When we observe that the superior speaker can charge air in such a brief period, we also must note that rapid air-charge should be mastered by all speakers. Here is the basis for reasonably effective performance. Only a few syllables per charge would be normal for most speakers. It appears to be easier to learn to take air in quickly than to take it in in large amounts. The very superior speaker probably does both, but by definition he is an exception to the rule.

Chapter VI

Acoustical Measurement and Pitch Perception in Alaryngeal Speech

E. THAYER CURRY

Background on Fundamental Vocal Frequency and Pitch Perception

W HEN CRITICALLY EVALUATED, many of the literature references to "pitch" are obviously concerned with "frequency." The frequency, as well as the relative sound pressure of an auditory stimulus can be measured in the complete absence of, and independently of, any listener. "Frequency" should be thought of as a distinctly physical attribute of the auditory stimulus; the unit is the Hertz. On the other hand, "pitch" as well as loudness is an auditory experience identified with the listener. "Pitch" should be thought of as the listener's personal auditory reaction to the acoustical or pure frequency stimulus; the unit is the mel. For a more complete evaluation of this psychophysical problem, the reader is referred to the pertinent discussion by Licklider (733). The following passage from van den Berg (62) is a rather typical example of usage for the term "pitch":

> Generally, the pitch of esophageal speech is rather low, between 50 and 100 Hz, on account of the rather large mass of the vibrating pseudolarynx. Occasionally, however, this mass is smaller and a more agreeable pitch results. The relations between the original properties of the structures, the type of operation, the method of training and the resulting pseudolarynx are not yet clearly established. The best results are observed when the ultimate structure is rather thin and pointed . . . .

Experimental Measures of Vocal Fundamental Frequency Levels and Fundamental Frequency Variability

The available experimental studies permit comment about several aspects of fundamental vocal frequency and formant amplitude as measured among alaryngeal speakers. The most remarkable physical aspect of the alaryngeal voice is, of course, the fundamental component of the vocal frequency. This parameter can be examined as to its (1) gross level in Hertz, (2) the range of frequencies spoken (i.e., the number of tones between the highest and lowest single frequencies utilized), (3) the standard deviation (SD) expressing the frequency variability, and (4) a somewhat more meaningful measure of range called the "90% range." Very recent (1967) data provide measures of format location and formant amplitude.

Table I presents some physical measures of frequency usage among alaryngeal speakers from studies by Damsté (151), Snidecor and Curry (708), Shipp (684), and Rollin (625). Unfortunately, these studies cited do not provide sufficient data to present a complete table. The frequency data taken from Damsté's Figure 5 have been contrasted with similar measures from the other indicated studies. Damsté's twenty subjects apparently had a median frequency of 67.5 Hz as an average for the group. This value is very close to the 63.3 Hz measure from Snidecor and Curry and to the mean value of 65.6 Hz from Rollin. Shipp's comparable frequency value is considerably higher for his comparable speaker group and will be considered separately.

The "usual pitch" of 60 per cent of the Damsté patients occurred in the four tone intervals which contained the median frequency values for all of the Snidecor and Curry subjects. The remaining 40 per cent of the Damsté patients were equally distributed, 20 per cent above and 20 per cent below the experimental group of Snidecor and Curry. However, the individual Damsté patients showed a much wider range of frequency usage than did the Snidercor and Curry subjects. The highest "usual" frequency estimated for any of the Damsté speakers was 185 Hz; this value compares with 80.8 Hz for the highest median frequency measured for any one of the Snidecor and Curry speakers. Actually, the highest frequency measured for any one of the Snidecor and Curry subjects was 135.5 Hz; this value is a half octave lower than the usual "pitch" for Damsté's patient number 21. It should be emphasized that the Snidecor and Curry speakers comprised a highly selected and homogeneous group which did not contain any pharyngeal speakers. The lowest frequency measured in this selected group was 17.2 Hz. Moreover, the tape recordings for all the six individuals in this group contained readily measurable periodicity in the octave between C_0 and C_1, that is, between 16.35 Hz and 32.70 Hz.

Selected data from Shipp's study (speakers designated as "the 6 best of a group of 33 speakers") indicate a significantly higher mean level of frequency usage, namely, 94.38 Hz. This is nearly four tones above the general level near 64 Hz as found in the studies by Damsté, Snidecor and Curry, and Rollin. Shipp suggests that these differences in fundamental frequency may be attributable to differences in the technique of analysis.

As a generalization, the combined data from Damsté, Snidecor and Curry, and Rollin would appear to substantiate the conclusion from Snidecor and Curry that the mean frequency level for most alaryngeal speakers is almost exactly one full octave below the level for the superior adult laryngeal speakers reported by Pronovost (200). This contrast in the frequency levels for the two groups is graphically presented in Figure 30.

Figure 30 presents graphic distributions of the frequencies measured for two groups of speakers (one laryngeal, one alaryngeal); each group had been rated as "superior" in a carefully controlled judgmental procedure. Although the forms of the two distributions are quite similar, the most obvious difference is, of course, the octave difference in the median frequency levels for the contrasted groups.

Measures of Formant Region Location and Formant Amplitude

Rollin (625) has estimated the center points for formants one, two, and three in comparable groups of laryngeal and alaryngeal speakers. His laryngeal speakers used a mean fundamental vocal frequency of 125 Hz compared with 65.6 Hz for a comparable group of alaryngeal speakers utilizing the same reading material. For all of the ten alaryngeal speakers of Rollin's study, center points for formants one and three were slightly higher than for the laryngeal speakers. In considering formant two, eight of the ten vowels of the study had a higher center point for the alaryngeal speakers. Rollin states: "For all of the esophageal subjects each of the lower three formants was located, and the task of locating these formants was easier than that involved in locating those of the normal speakers."

The coordinate plots illustrating formants one and two covered larger areas for the vowels of the alaryngeal speakers than for

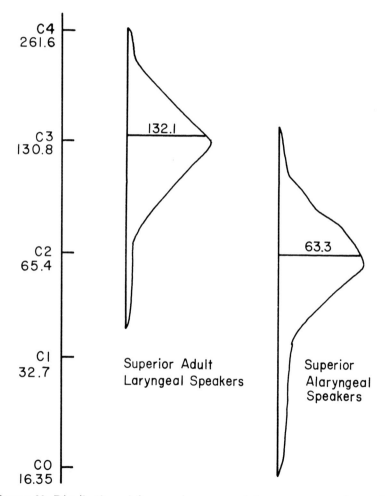

FIGURE 30. Distribution of frequencies measured for two groups of superior speakers. Great variability for both classes of speakers and almost exactly an octave difference in average pitch level are shown.

the laryngeal speakers of the study. Rollin felt that the alaryngeal speakers might find difficulty in making the fine adjustments in the articulatory mechanism necessary to create more restricted vowel formant areas. As we will see later, the intelligibility measures for Rollin's alaryngeal subjects were adversely influenced, very probably by this inexactness among the vowel formant regions. The amplitude of formants one, two, and three for most vowels was greater among Rollin's alaryngeal subjects than for his comparable laryngeal speakers.

Fundamental Vocal Frequency and Variability as Measured with Superior Alaryngeal Speakers

Snidecor and Curry (708)) have described their experimental results with carefully selected alaryngeal subjects judged to be reading a standard passage in a highly superior manner. The measurements of fundamental vocal frequency were obtained by utilizing the phonophotographic technique described by Cowan (135). The temporal extent of each measurement interval was 0.051 seconds. The average reading time, 28.3 seconds for the entire passage, was utilized as follows:

Silence: 38.5 per cent

Aperiodic sound: 1.9 per cent

Clearly periodic fundamental vocal frequency: 59.6 per cent

TABLE I
MEASURES OF FUNDAMENTAL VOCAL FREQUENCY USAGE

	Damste	Snidecor & Curry	Shipp*	Rollin
	(1958)	(1961)	(1967)	(1967)
Fundamental frequency				
Mean (in Hz)			94.38	65.6
Median (in Hz)	67.5	63.3	86.1	
SD (in tones)		2.30	2.56	
90% range (in tones)		6.5	8.25	
Highest frequency (in Hz)	(185?)	135.5		
Lowest frequency (in Hz)		17.2		

*Values for six best speakers. This group should be compared with the six selected superior speakers in Snidecor and Curry's study.

TABLE II
MEASURES OF FUNDAMENTAL FREQUENCY IN EXPERIMENTAL
GROUP OF SUPERIOR ALARYNGEAL SPEAKERS

Measured Frequency Interval (in Hz)	Speakers of Snidecor-Curry Study						Group Total
	1	*3*	*5*	*7*	*8*	*6*	
130.81–146.80	1						1
116.51–130.80	5	2	2				9
103.81–116.50	17		4	1	2		24
92.51–103.80	61	5	21	1	15	2	105
82.41– 92.50	67	6	30	1	30	8	142
73.44– 82.40	63M*	30	64	37	64	23	281
65.41– 73.43	33	54	62M*	64	78M*	34	325
58.27– 65.40	30	93M*	73	58	80	63	397M*
51.92– 58.26	10	73	46	63M*	37	56M	285
46.26– 51.91	11	42	19	49	15	54*	190
41.21– 46.25	14	9	15	27	6	44	115
36.72– 41.20	4	5	9	15	1	19	53
32.71– 36.71	3	1	5	6	2	13	30
29.12– 32.70	1	1	1	1		3	7
25.96– 29.11			1	1	3	5	10
23.12– 25.95				1	1	2	4
20.60– 23.11						3	3
18.35– 20.59					1		1
16.36– 18.34						1	1
Total periodic intervals	320	321	352	325	335	330	1983
Aperiodic intervals	1	4	4	6	44	4	63
Silence	254	157	165	219	234	253	1282
Total intervals	575	482	521	550	613	587	3328

M—Median frequency interval.
*Mean frequency interval.

Table II presents a distribution of the fundamental frequency measures for the group of superior alaryngeal speakers. Variations among the individual subjects, as well as central tendencies for the group, are readily observed. The distribution of frequencies used by this superior group has been plotted and previously presented in Figure 30. Additional measures of frequency range and variability are tabulated in Table III. The frequency value in Hz for the highest and lowest measurable periodic interval is

TABLE III
MEASURES OF FREQUENCY RANGE OF SUPERIOR
ALARYNGEAL SPEAKER GROUP

Shortest measurable	Speakers					
periodic interval	1	3	5	7	8	6
Frequency	135.5	123.4	118.7	112.3	106.6	95.2
Tones above 16.35 (Hz)	18.3	17.5	17.2	16.7	16.2	15.2
Longest measurable						
periodic interval						
Frequency (Hz)	32.2	30.4	28.3	24.0	19.5	17.2
Tones above 16.35 (Hz)	5.9	5.4	4.8	3.3	1.5	4.0
Total range of						
frequency measured						
Tones	12.4	12.1	12.4	14.8	13.4	14.7
Octaves	2.1	2.0	2.1	2.5	2.2	2.5
"Effective range"						
median 90%						
Tones	7.8	4.7	7.2	6.1	6.0	7.2
Octaves	1.3	0.8	1.2	1.1	1.0	1.2
Median frequency						
In Hz	80.8	60.4	66.2	58.2	67.3	54.0
Tones above 16.35 Hz	13.8	11.3	12.2	11.0	12.3	10.4
Mean frequency						
In Hz	76.7	60.5	65.8	57.3	66.7	50.9
Tones above 16.35 Hz	13.4	11.3	12.1	10.9	12.2	9.7

TABLE IV
EXTENTS, DIRECTIONS, AND RATES OF FREQUENCY
MOVEMENT DURING SPEECH OF SUPERIOR
ALARYNGEAL SUBJECTS

Frequency change during inflections	Up	Down	Total
Number	275	309	584
Per cent of total number	47	53	100
Mean extent in tones	2.0	2.8	2.4
Mean rate of frequency movement*			7.9
Frequency change during shifts	Up	Down	Total
Number	121	54	175
Per cent of total number	69	31	100
Mean extent in tones	3.1	2.0	2.8
Mean rate of frequency movement*			4.3

shown for each of the six subjects. The total range, in tones and in octaves, between the highest and lowest frequency is indicated for each superior speaker. A somewhat more meaningful value, the median 90 per cent of frequencies produced, or the "effective range," is greater than one octave for five of the six superior subjects under study.

The extent, direction, and rate of frequency movements during the speech of superior alaryngeal subjects is indicated in Table IV. Inflections are frequency movements during vocalizations; shifts are frequency movements between vocalizations. Both laryngeal and alaryngeal speaker groups have the same predominant pattern of frequency movement during speech: downward by means of inflections and upward by means of shifts. For the alaryngeal speaker group, 53 per cent of the inflections were downward with a mean extent of 2.8 tones. On the other hand, 69 per cent of the shifts were upward and had a mean extent of 3.1 tones. The rate of frequency movement was 7.9 tones per second during inflections and 4.3 tones per second during shifts.

Pitch Perception and Vowel Intelligibility

The fundamental frequency vocalizations of the alaryngeal speaker are produced in a frequency range which has special perception problems. These rather obvious perceptual aspects of alaryngeal speech (*i.e.* the "pitch" aspects) have been considered by many authors. A passage from van den Berg (62) is of particular pertinence:

> The variations in pitch which can be produced by the patient are much more limited than those which can be made in laryngeal speech. The reasons are obvious. In the larynx we have a very complicated (sic) and delicate complex of muscles which allow for compensatory mechanisms, while in the pseudolarynx only one muscle is present.

Damsté recognizes this problem and discusses the acoustic properties of alaryngeal speaking as follows:

> The fundamental tone of an oesophageal voice is often difficult to determine. This is because the frequency is low and because the sound is very complex, in other words the fundamental tone is accompanied by a large number of relatively strong overtones. The ear is not very sensitive in the frequency range of the partials. And the latter contain a large part of the total sound-energy.

Damsté's observation regarding the relative insensitiveness of the human ear at the frequency range of the fundamental of the alaryngeal speakers has been indicated by the work of Rollin. to frequency and pitch in this low-frequency region. Stevens and Volkmann's curve (734), which clearly shows this perceptual-physical relation, has very important practical implications for the alaryngeal speaker who is attempting to improve his speaking performance by increasing the frequency variability of his pseudo-laryngeal output. The perceptual problem is clearly shown by the data of Snidecor and Curry. Their study found a mean total frequency range of 13.21 tones (variability around a mean of 63.3 Hz) for the superior alaryngeal speakers and only 10.5 tones (however, variability about a mean of 132.1 Hz) for superior adult speakers with normal laryngeal function. In spite of this greater frequency variability measured for the alaryngeal speakers, this group was nonetheless judged to have a "restricted pitch range" when the tape recordings were perceptually evaluated. The physical measures indicated a considerably greater frequency movement than was apparent in pitch to the listener. This lack of agreement between measured frequency and the pitch aspects of these low-frequency speaking performances can readily be understood from Stevens and Volkmann's experiment.

Another factor contributing to the "poor perception" of these alaryngeal speakers has been indicated by the work of Rollin. The greater variability of vowel formants one and two, resulting in the physical overlap of adjacent vowels among alaryngeal speakers, considerably reduced the vowel intelligibility measured in the speaking performance of this group. The nonoverlapping of vowels among the laryngeal speakers doubtless accounted for the higher intelligibility scores in this group.

The alaryngeal speaker should continuously be encouraged to extend the range of frequencies produced in his speaking performances. However, because of the particular frequency-pitch relationship which functions in the fundamental frequency region of alaryngeal speech, the extensions of frequency range will not be as productive of perceptual variability as would be readily apparent in the higher-frequency regions characteristic of the normal laryngeal speaking range. Also, the alaryngeal speaker should be highly encouraged to make every effort to sharpen his articulatory precision. Such efforts should increase his vowel intelligibility and the consequent overall comprehension of his speaking.

Increasing Fundamental Frequency Variability

The work of van den Berg discusses certain aspects of increasing the frequency variability of alaryngeal speech:

Therefore, pitch and intensity are correlated in oesophageal speech. A low pitch is produced with a low intensity of the voice, a high pitch with a high intensity. This increase of the pitch at increasing intensity, i.e., at increasing flow of air through the pseudoglottis, is caused by the Bernoulli effect of the air which escapes through the narrow opening. The walls are sucked towards each other by the negative pressure in the pseudoglottis and this effect increases the effective stiffness of the muscular structures, which then vibrate at a high frequency, as their mass remains the same.

The speech of a clever patient sometimes gives the illusion of agreeable changes of pitch which objectively are not present [sic]. He uses his vocal cavities in such a way that the resonant frequencies, or formants, change during the pronunciation of the vowel in question. Occasionally, the range of tensions in the region of the pseudolarynx is very small. The range of pitches may then be improved by exerting an additional pressure, e.g., by means of a finger, by compressing the neck against a collar or by bending the head downwards. A well designed collar may be very useful when the crico-pharyngeal sphincter, or what is left of it, is so weak that the oesophageal air escapes at such a low pressure that the intensity of the voice is too low.

In another work, van den Berg (63) shows vowel constant spectra with clear variation in frequency accompanying pressure variations.

Thus, the pitch is secondary compared with the intensity and the subject had to make himself clear about how to produce the high pitch. Therefore, he always separated the section with a high pitch from that with a low pitch by a new breath and a new injection of air into the oesophagus.

The relationship between pitch and intensity is clearly shown in Hyman's training recordings contained in the lesson on stress. Specific suggestions for drill on pitch variability are given in Chapter VIII.

Another result of Shipp's research is of especial importance in retraining the alaryngeal voice. Shipp's study clearly indicated that alaryngeal speakers with higher fundamental vocal frequency usage (as described by higher mean values) obtained greater acceptability ratings from his listening group. This significant finding should be used to encourage surgeons, therapists, and patients to provide the optimum conditions for as high a postoperative fundamental vocal frequency as possible.

Chapter VII

Loudness and Quality in Esophageal Speech and the Artificial Larynx

ALAN C. NICHOLS

T HE FIRST GOAL OF an esophageal speaker is the control of voice which leads to fluency. The second goal is intelligibility, an achievement that is even closer to the basic requirements for communication than simple fluency. When a command of fluency and intelligibility in common circumstances is achieved, the temptation to stop working on voice improvement is often irresistible.

Experience indicates, however, that even excellent speakers improve their voices with practice when their goals are realistic. Two of these goals are (1) greater loudness and (2) better voice quality. The present chapter presents a synthesis of clinical and theoretical information for establishing realistic goals for the improvement of loudness and quality.

Loudness

Only the rare esophageal speaker can "turn up the volume" of his voice so that he can project to everyone in a room, or overcome the noise of a hallway, a busy street, or a room full of running machines. All of these situations are common in business and social life, that is to say, situations in which the esophageal speaker intends to use his voice.

The process of turning up the volume on a radio is an appropriate analogy to increasing the loudness of a voice. However, the analogy is not perfect. Loudness, from the listener's point of view, is complex — a function of the relative levels of pitch and intensity, and of the current condition of his hearing and attention. The low pitch of the typical esophageal voice, for example, is harder to hear and amplify than the ordinary voice.

The present discussion, unless otherwise specified, will employ the term "loudness" in the sense of the apparent power of the speaker.

Other factors being equal, the harder the air is forced through the pseudoglottis, the louder the voice will be. Strother (741) remarks, "Exercises used for increasing loudness [in the esophageal voice] are similar to those used with normal voices, e.g., the production of tones of increasing loudness, starting with the softest tone the patient can produce." He adds that increasing loudness has one great drawback — forcing almost inevitably produces tension that may lead to soreness and irritation, and consequently to a slowing or stopping of progress. For example, Genereux (252) found in her "pilot study" of an esophageal speaker that increasing loudness led to poorer quality.

A procedure that may minimize artificial tensions has been suggested by Drummond (180). She found that practice in a noisy environment — she used "white" noise in her initial studies — improved loudness and intelligibility. Later experiences of rejection of "white" noise by clients led her to use music as a masking source (181). More study of esophageal voice practice in noisy environments, and perhaps even under conditions of delayed feedback (813), may lead to techniques of high utility where the increase of the loudness of an esophageal speaker is concerned. Drummond (181) points out that home practice is possible with "transistor radio music close to the ear," which makes such practice readily available. It should be noted that the production of loudness without excess tension is always the goal. A judicial adjustment of the loudness of the noise source should always be considered if struggle is noted.

While the weakness of the voice may be due to the lack of force in the expelled air, the strength and control of the involved muscles is critical. If the speaker has developed strong muscles with integrated control, the problem of maintaining muscular coordination is greatly lessened and the production of louder tones becomes possible. Thus, most authorities suggest that the pupil delay work on loudness until a late period of therapy. Mary Doehler (176) has contributed the following:

> Up to this point, I have said very little in relation to volume because, personally I feel that it is more important first to gain control and develop correct habits of articulation. When I feel the pupil is gaining

control, I suggest the following exercises: In a low tone, but not in a whisper, say "one." Then as loudly as possible repeat "one." This will require careful scrutiny on the part of the teacher, in order to note that there is not facial contraction, extra motions of the body, or a strained throat . . . another exercise is the ladder exercise, where each ascending step of the ladder is a louder tone . . . every laryngectomized patient should be able to call "Fire!" in a loud tone.

Mrs. Doehler's goal for the esophageal speaker, "Fire!" in a loud voice, is encouraging. This goal, however, is questionable as a realistic objective for all speakers. In order to discuss the point, the physical bases of loudness in the esophageal voice should be clarified.

Study of the discussion of the pseudoglottis in Chapter IV will reveal that the sound of the esophageal voice is produced by the vibration of some portion of the esophagus or pharynx. Air is stored behind this area by one of the three methods described in Chapter XI and, in being forced out through the constriction, produces the series of puffs that are heard as voiced speech sounds. Two factors are considered in a discussion of the loudness of the sound produced at the pseudoglottis: the *mass* and *elasticity* of the tissues involved.

The mass of the tissues makes possible the buildup of air pressure behind the pseudoglottis — little pressure or power, and therefore little loudness, could be held behind a light barrier. In addition, the tissues must be elastic to open, emit a puff of air, and return to a closed position as the pressure drops.

It is obvious that the volume of air behind the pseudoglottis must be sufficient to continue this sequence, or voice ceases. The necessary and sufficient air volumes for esophageal speakers have been discussed by Isshiki and Snidecor (356).

The variety of levels in speech produced by esophageal and normal speakers is illustrated in the sonagrams in Figure 31. At the tops of the sonagrams labeled A, B, and C, the pressures of phrases spoken by a normal speaker and by high-rated and low-rated esophageal speakers are displayed. The scale to the right of the pressure plots was calibrated in terms of decibels with reference to the base line. The vowels are discernibly important to loudness in both the normal and esophageal speakers. Note the amplitude pattern of the word "long," as produced by the high-rated esophageal speaker. The prolonged vowel *aw*, the *o* in "long," shows the fluctuating pressure as the pseudoglottis emits puffs of air. The same effect is notable in other vowels produced by this speaker. Snidecor and Isshiki (709) report similar fluctuations for their superior esophageal speaker. The effect is not as prominent in the amplitude display of the normal speaker because of the relatively higher frequency of emission of air puffs.

Under the pseudoglottis, there must also be a muscular or elastic force producing the pressure on the charged air. This force, Damsté (151) attributes to two sources: (1) the natural elasticity of esophageal tissues forced apart by the charge of air and (2) intratracheal pressures on the esophagus produced by the increased force of breathing which Damsté asserts accompanies loud speech in the esophageal voice. The former mechanism, he states, is effective for the speaker using the injection method for relatively quiet speech; the speaker using the suction method is limited to the latter mechanism.

A notable application of Damsté's principles by a laryngectomee is the action taken by J.L.R., an executive with considerable speaking force. In a situation in which he feels the need for greater loudness, he protrudes his chin, elongates his neck and the underlying phonation mechanism, and consequently adds greatly to the natural elasticity of the area about the reservoir of air. The effect is a louder voice — a voice, according to his wife, that is capable of "yelling upstairs to get his daughter out of the bathroom in the morning."

The mass of the tissues of the pseudoglottis is dependent upon the anatomy of the speaker before laryngectomy and upon the extent and nature of the operation. (See Pressman's discussion at this point.) The elasticity of the tissues has similar determinants, as do the strength and tonus of the muscles of phonation. Practice can improve the control and the strength needed for a louder voice, but mass and elasticity of the tissues of the speaker's phonating mechanisms may preclude a voice of sufficient loudness to yell, "Fire!"

The relative loudness of the esophageal voice and the normal voice has been studied by Hyman (343). His speakers included eight who had normal voices and eight who used esophageal voice. The peak intensity levels he reports as approximate measures of their loudness levels were 79 dB (normal) and 73 dB (esophageal). A more recent study by Snidecor and Isshiki (711), using different equipment and procedures, provides the following information: their superior esophageal speaker was able to produce an *ah* at an instantaneous 85 dB level, as contrasted with the 95 dB of a normal speaker. The comparable loudness ranges of esophageal and normal voices may be exemplified by data from several sources. Fletcher (212) reported a range of over 21 dB for telephone conversations, which provides an estimate of the functional midrange of intensities among normal speakers. Hyman (343) found the average intensity range of his eight esophageal speakers to be 11 dB. A first approximation of the contrasting limits of loudness for normal and esophageal speakers is provided by Snidecor and Isshiki (711). They found that a normal speaker made smooth intensity changes which ranged up to 45 dB. Their superior esophageal speaker managed a range of 20 dB.

For those whose esophageal voices are too soft, other resources are available. One such is the artificial larynx. The Hyman (343) study showed that the reed-type artificial larynx, no longer available, was often louder than the normal voice under controlled conditions. With the electronic larynx, loudness is a matter of adjusting the power to an adequate level or buying a more powerful instrument. Barney, Haworth, and Dunn (34) studied this problem at some length. The loudness of the artificial larynx they developed was felt adequate for conversational purposes although, in situations in which the normal speaker would increase his intensity, they advised that the speaker move closer to his listener. The vowel peaks with this instrument approximated 70 to 75 dB re .0002 dynes per cm^2 at a distance of three feet.

Greene (280) reports that artificial larynges should be tried out by a client, for each speaker has different needs. She writes, "After extensive experimentation we retain the Western Electric

Mark 5,™ the Aurex Neovox,™ and the Dutch . . . DSP-8.™ . . . By far the most successful and popular is the Aurex."

One more electronic device should be noted: the small hand microphone and loudspeaker (such as the one listed in the Appendix, "Directory of Sources of Supply,") used by some speakers to increase the loudness of their speech. This device can supply a useful increase in loudness when the speaker must talk in a noisy office or restaurant, in a small group, and so forth. It will save a great deal of effort for those who constantly use their esophageal voices. Greene (280) suggests from clinical experience that amplifiers may improve confidence, relax the speaker, and enable him to evaluate his voice more objectively. In this sense, she remarks it may be "a valuable teaching aid." However, she adds that some speakers' voices may be too low in pitch to amplify.

Finally, consideration should be given to the relationship between the actual magnitude of the voice and the apparent loudness of the voice as a function of the speaker's intelligibility. The intelligibile voice need not be as loud as the unintelligible voice to be comfortable for the listener. Consequently, an improvement in intelligibility may provide an apparent increase in loudness. The tendency of some speakers to finish words, sentences, and phrases in a whisper rather than charge more air behind the pseudoglottis also has an effect on apparent loudness. These speakers are usually beginners who have not developed voluntary control of their esophageal voices. Experienced speakers learn to adjust their rates to achieve control.

Quality

One young esophageal speaker from Columbus, Ohio, tells the following story with a great deal of enjoyment:

> One day I ran into an old friend. We talked awhile, and then he said, "You have a really bad cold, don't you?" "No, brother," I said, "I haven't had a cold in a year." "But you're losing your voice, aren't you?" "I just got it back three months ago," I said, "I had my larynx taken out last fall, and I'm lucky to have a voice at all."

The situation described in this anecdote is fairly common. In an incident related by Shryock (687), the confused listener was a physician. "I can tell by your voice," said the doctor, "that you are developing laryngitis and I advise you to do something to take care of yourself." "Well, doctor," he [the esophageal speaker] replied, "you must be mistaken, I haven't any larynx."

These incidents serve to show that the vocal quality of the esophageal speaker is different from the quality of the normal voice. His voice is often hoarse, and he is frequently thought to have a cold.

The term "quality" is not consistently defined. The term has been used as a synonym for "general effectiveness." A narrower definition is made by speech pathologists and phoneticians. Their usage is synonymous with "timbre" and is limited to the psycho-acoustic effect of the harmonic structure of the voice.

Fairbanks (200) made the following explanation of the bases of quality: "Voice quality is a property of all voiced intervals, but is significant primarily during vowels. Its sources of variation lie in the generation of the vocal fold tone and in the transmission of the tone through the vocal channel."

In relating this explanation to esophageal voice, two considerations should be noted. First, the generation of the voice in the esophageal speaker is dependent upon the pseudoglottis, not the vocal folds. Second, when the operation removes only the larynx, the transmission of the tone through the vocal channel is probably not changed greatly. Rollin (625), however, found that the mean frequencies of the first three vowel formants, particularly the second and third, were significantly higher for esophageal speakers than for normal speakers. This was true even though the fundamental frequencies of the normal speakers were significantly higher. These results would suggest that the esophageal speaker forms smaller resonators in his oral cavity with his tongue. Power-level integration spectra of the "before" and "after" laryngectomy speech of an esophageal speaker made by Nichols (542) tend to confirm the Rollin findings. The same speaker's normal voice showed higher fundamentals than his later esophageal voice, but his esophageal voice tended to have higher-frequency overtones. On the basis of these observations, it might be hypothesized that the esophageal speaker carries his tongue higher. Perry's (587) dissertation lends support to this hypothesis. He found that the fundamental frequency does not change from vowel to vowel in esophageal speakers as it does in normal speech. He hypothesized that the base of the tongue is freed from the vocal source by the laryngectomy. Thus, tongue adjustment for the vowels does not alter the frequency of the vocal source. Such freedom from lower structures might also contribute to carrying the tongue higher in the oral cavity with the effect on harmonics noted above. Study of the effects of more open vowel articulations on the voice quality and intelligibility of the esophageal speaker may prove fruitful.

Notwithstanding the suggestions in recent studies that vowel articulation may be affected by the operation, it is at the level of the generation of the voice that the primary sources of differences in the esophageal voice may be found.

Particular attention should be paid to Fairbanks' comment that quality is primarily a characteristic of the vowels. Vowels are differentiated from one another by their harmonic characteristics, and these harmonic compositions are produced largely by adjustments of the resonating cavities of the oral mechanism. This observation leads to the conclusion that careful articulation of the vowels in speaking should have a beneficial effect on the quality of the voice. This can be achieved by concentrating on making the vowels discriminately different from one another — to put it another way, by concentration on intelligibility. In addition, practice in giving each vowel its full duration, and the acquisition of relaxed control of vowel production, may prove helpful. The nonsense-syllable drill proposed by Doehler (176) with her insistence that the final vowel be "finished," that is, given its full duration, is one example of the many procedures for developing a mastery of the vowels.

Fairbanks (200) described four types of voice quality disorders: harshness, breathiness, and hoarseness, which he identified as defects of tone generation; and nasality, a defect of transmission. The quality defect most frequently noted in the voice of the esophageal speaker is similar to hoarseness. Fairbanks' discussion follows:

Universally familiar as a symptom of acute laryngitis, hoarseness combines the features of harshness and breathiness . . . . Irregular aperiodic noise in the vocal fold spectrum is the distinguishing feature of harshness. A common cause is excessive laryngeal tension . . . . In breathy quality the vocal folds vibrate, but the intermittent closure fails and airflow is continuous. The firmness of the basic glottal closure is insufficient for a given airflow (or the force of the airflow is excessive for a given closure). Breathy quality is almost invariably accompanied by limited vocal intensity . . . .

One procedure for quantifying Fairbanks' categories for experimental and clinical purposes is the development of rating scales. The equal-appearing interval scales of Paddock (569), for example, allow the listener to match unknown voice samples to scaled samples that represent rated levels of severity of harshness, breathiness, and hoarseness. The scales provide a seven-point range, "one" being indicative of "good voice" and "seven" indicating "poorest voice." To illustrate, the pseudovoices resulting from two Asai-type operations (11, 12) were compared to the esophageal voices of two "good" and two "beginning" esophageal speakers. The results were as follows in Table I.

TABLE I
VOICE QUALITY RATINGS FOR SPEAKERS USING
THE ASAI AND ESOPHAGEAL VOICES

	(Paddock scales) *		
	Harshness	*Breathiness*	*Hoarseness*
Asai speakers			
Male			
One Month	4.9	2.9	5.5
Three Months	5.7	5.1	6.3
Four Months	5.3	6.8	6.7
Female	6.1	6.5	6.8
Esophageal speakers			
Male 2 Beginner	6.3	2.0	6.7
Male 3 Beginner	6.8	2.3	6.9
Male 4 Good	6.1	3.1	6.5
Male 5 Good	6.3	2.9	6.8

The use of the Paddock scales, which were developed for scaling the defectiveness of the normal voice, place a procedural limitation on the conclusions that may be drawn from the ratings. With this in mind, it is still notable that the harshness ratings indicate a better vocal quality for the Asai voice. The hoarseness ratings do not show clear-cut differences. The growth of the breathiness ratings for the male Asai speaker over the months in which he was acquiring control over his voice and the female speaker's breathiness are striking. It may be inferred that less complete closure of the pseudoglottis was made as the voice developed, producing that turbulent airflow which results in broad-band noise acoustically. A discussion of such effects in the pathological larynx is provided by Yanagihara (825). The source of the breathiness is less obvious than its mechanics. Stiffening tissues or struggle may both be involved. Moments of failure of phonation may be noted in the recordings of the speech of the two Asai speakers and, from the clinical point of view, tension is a prominent characteristic of the Asai speakers' vocal productions. It would be premature to base conclusions on the speech of two clients, but areas for further study have been identified.

The sources of vocal quality deviations in the esophageal voice are complex. In the pictures prepared by Rubin, presented earlier in Figure 26, it will be noted that mucus has collected at the pseudoglottis. Although limited amounts of mucus may collect on the vocal folds of the normal speaker without apparent effect on the quality of the voice, greater amounts collect with the advent of respiratory infections. Vibration of the mucus contributes to irregular, aperiodic noise in the spectrum of the normal or esophageal voice. Damsté (151) placed a great deal of importance on the surgical formation of a pseudoglottis above any diverticula which may serve to collect mucus. He noted that five out of eight poor voices studied could be seen by x-ray photography to have a pouch in the anterior pharyngeal wall, above or at the level of the pseudoglottis, with an accumulation of mucus. In the normal larynx, mucus is cleared from the vocal source by coughing. For the esophageal speaker, swallowing does not appear to be as effective a mechanism for this purpose. However, as Damsté has demonstrated, it is possible to change the site of the pseudoglottis in some cases, raising it above the diverticula. Cold and hot drinks may also serve to clear the esophagus of excess mucus.

Still another cause of hoarseness may be the structures involved in the pseudoglottis itself. Diedrich (174) points out that the pseudoglottis is a long sphincter in the superior speaker. Its length may be from 10 to 20 mm and may, in certain cases, extend to 28 or 30 mm. The tissues of the pseudoglottis are not inserted in cartilage as are the vocal folds; the maintenance of tension, consequently, is less controlled; and the vibration pattern is more complex. Along the length of the sphincter, certain sections may contribute vibrations at least partially independent of the overall pattern of vibration. Scar tissue and discontinuity of muscle tissues may contribute to irregular vibratory patterns. Irregularities in the movements and conformation of the pseudoglottis itself probably produce noisy turbulence. Tension adds to such irregularities. Yanagihara's (825) discussion of the hoarseness experienced by normal speakers has been mentioned. He adds: "Loss of high frequency components may be attributable to the incomplete or shorter closing phase during vibratory cycles." Similar observations may apply to the pseudoglottis. Studies of the closing phase and opening quotient of the pseudoglottis may prove fruitful. Luchsinger and Arnold (453) provide discussions of these measures and their theoretical implications for vocal production. It may be concluded that the continuous elasticity of the tissues involved is dependent upon the nature and results of the operation in conjunction with the tension and struggle of the speaker. The operation itself determines much of the characteristic quality of the esophageal voice.

Shipp (684) has also pointed out that acceptability of esophageal voice is affected significantly by respiratory noise. Apparently, the average listener does not have much tolerance for the masking noise that comes from breathing in conjunction with the production of esophageal voice. Notwithstanding the contributions of simultaneous breathing to vocal production and loudness, then, the reduction of such noise to a minimum will have desirable effects upon the listener's impressions of vocal quality.

Figures 31 and 32 show sonagrams of a normal voice and two esophageal voices. Sonagram A of Figure 31 shows a normal speaker saying the phrase, "These take the shape of a long round arch."

The frequency of the vocal pattern is shown on the vertical dimension; time is shown on the horizontal dimension. The dark horizontal areas on the sonagram are called bars or formants and represent the harmonics of the vocal tone. The differences in harmonic structure across the sonagram were produced by the speaker's adjustments of his oral structures and are interpreted by a listener as the different vowels and diphthongs of the language. The relative darkness of the trace indicates the loudness of the frequencies represented.

Inspection of the three sections of Figure 31, the broad-band spectrograms, shows that the formants of normal speech are clearly formed, that several formants occur below 5000 Hz and that in general the areas outside of the formants are clean (i.e. free of noise). The vertical striations of the normal speaker, roughly equivalent to the movements of the vocal folds, are regular in contrast to the irregular striations of the esophageal speakers. However, according to Barney, Haworth, and Dunn (34), too regular a pattern such as that produced by the artificial larynx is also an undesirable characteristic to a listener. Although the speaker in sonagram B of Figure 31 was a high-rated esophageal speaker, the contrasts between his spectrogram and the tracing of the normal speaker are readily detectable. Particularly notable is the irregularity of the esophageal vibratory pattern. As Fairbanks (200) has noted, this is characteristic of the harsh, hoarse voice. These observations point out still another direction for therapy. Regularity of the vibratory pattern may be achieved by practice in prolonging vowels, striving for a relaxation consistent with effective intensity as well as duration. Brodnitz (92) suggests that "freedom for movement" may be a better metaphor than "relaxation" to describe to the learner the optimal muscle tone for vocal production. Teachers of esophageal voice may find his discussion of the semantics of voice therapy helpful. This practice is particularly important in the beginning when habits are being formed.

The lack of clearly defined harmonic structure in the esophageal speaker is also observable in the sonagrams. Damsté (151) asserts that the harmonic structure of the esophageal speaker is more complex than that of the normal speaker because the funda-

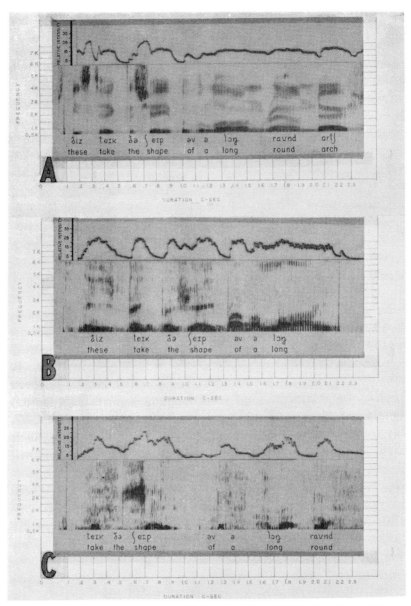

FIGURE 31. Broad-band sonagrams of three speakers saying the phrase "These take the shape of a long round arch." A. "Normal" speaker, B. "High-rated" esophageal speaker, C. "Low-rated" esophageal speaker. The trace at the top shows the power level of the speech during the production of the phrase. Note the relatively well-defined harmonic structure of the normal rated esophageal speaker's phrase, and the relative dominance of the random, inharmonic "noise" in the low-rated esophageal speaker's phrase.

mental is lower and the upper harmonics, consequently, closer together. This assertion would be more convincing if harmonics were clearly discernible in the sonagrams of esophageal speakers as they are in sonagrams of laryngeal voice. It is perhaps more accurate an appraisal of the sonagrams we have of esophageal voice to say that the harmonic aspects of the patterns are far outweighed by the inharmonic broad-band noise introduced by irregularities of vibration and consequent turbulence of the airflow. The formants of esophageal voice may then be understood as resonant emphases of selected narrow bands of this inharmonic broad-band noise. This interpretation of sonagraphic evidence may also apply to the Asai voices discussed earlier. On the other hand, better evidence of harmonic components does appear in sonagrams of these voices, particularly in the later months of development of the male voice. However, the broad-band noise is even more apparent in the developed Asai voice than in the beginning voice. Noise fills the whole spectrum and darkens the areas between the formants. This is the sonagraphic equivalent of the breathiness noted as characteristic of the Asai voice earlier.

So important is noise to hoarseness that Yanagihara (825) has been able to develop a reliable ordinal scaling of hoarse voices on the basis of sonagrams. For example, the speaker represented by sonagram B of Figure 32 would be classed as a type IV (severe hoarseness) on Yanagihara's scale. On the other hand, Snidecor and Isshiki's (711) superior speaker appears to shift from a type IV to a type II (moderate to slight hoarseness) on a perceptual scale, as he reduces his intensity. Damsté's (151) speaker appears to fall into the type IV category, but his broad-band sonagram is more difficult to relate to Yanagihara's schematic presentation. The Asai spectrograms are uniformly type IV.

It should be noted that both of the esophageal speakers represented by B and C of Figure 31 were understandable. The speaker in B was highly rated, even without the complex overtone structure of the normal voice, although he has more structure than the lowly rated esophageal speaker in C.

Figure 32 shows narrow-band sonagrams of the normal, the high-rated, and the low-rated esophageal speakers. The harmonic

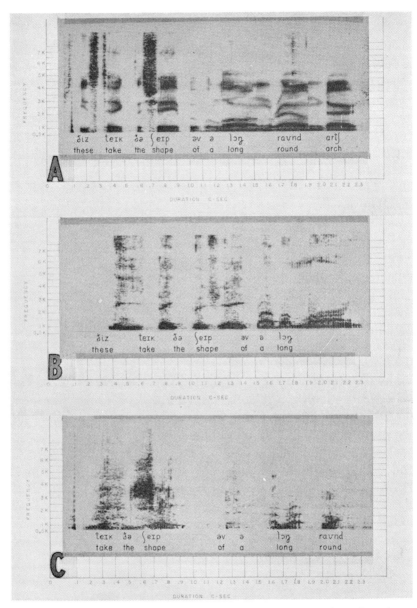

FIGURE 32. Narrow-band sonagrams of three speakers saying the phrase "These take the shape of a long round arch." A. "Normal" speaker, B. "High-rated" esophageal speaker, C. "Low-rated" esophageal speaker. Note the relatively powerful middle harmonics of the normal speaker, the presence of higher harmonics in the high-rated speaker's phrase, and the absence of middle and upper harmonics in the low-rated speaker's phrase.

structure of the normal speaker is more apparent in these displays. It is more difficult to distinguish the formant structure of the esophageal voices. Again the formants of the high-rated speaker are more clearly defined than those of the low-rated speaker. Other sonagrams of excellent speakers confirm this observation. In the best speakers, a formant structure very close to that of the normal voice may be noted on certain vowels. Waldrop and Toht's (796) frequency-amplitude displays of vowels may further illustrate this point. Figure 33 shows their analysis of the acoustic power of a vowel in relation to frequency as produced by a "normal" voice, a "pharyngeal" voice, and "esophageal" voice, and a "buccal whisper." It will be noted that the formants, shown here by the peaks of intensity, of the "pharyngeal" voice are more clearly defined and closer to the shape of the formants of the "normal" voice than those of the "esophageal" voice; and the formants of the "buccal whisper" are most undefined. Tape-recorded samples of the speech of these individuals demonstrate the superior quality of the "pharyngeal" speaker, and the poor intelligibility of the "buccal whisper." These observations tend to support the importance of practice for clearly defined vowel production mentioned at the beginning of this chapter.

In a general sense, references to effectiveness have some relevance to the topic of quality. For example, Levin (439) says that "the quality of speech depends upon early training after the operation." He also reports, "quality of the voice improves steadily for about three years, as has been proved by follow-up recordings." Three years, however, may be a conservative estimate. Discussions on this topic among laryngectomees often include comments that the speaker's voice has been improving for five, six, or seven years.

Quality, in the sense of timbre, may make an important contribution to the improvement noted by Levin. Damsté (151) says that the bases of quality are "purity of voice (probably timbre), intensity, velocity, phrasing and voice-melody." As has been pointed out, Shipp's (684) listeners felt that breathing noise was important to the "acceptability" of esophageal voice. He reports several other factors that were correlated with the rated accept-

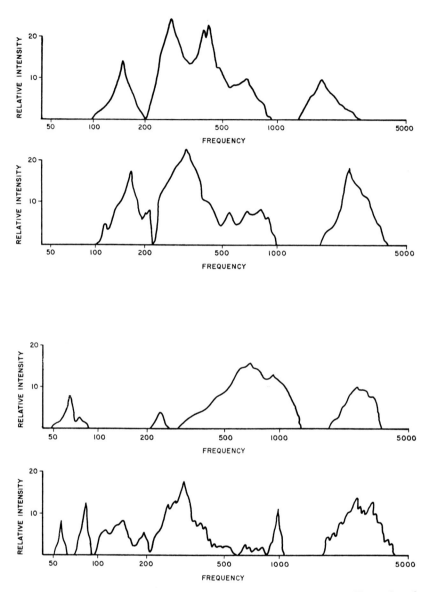

FIGURE 33. Power level versus frequency graphs of the vowel *e* [i] produced by four speakers: 1. "normal" laryngeal voice, 2. "pharyngeal" voice, 3. "esophageal" voice, 4. "buccal" voice. The graphs are tracings of results obtained by Waldrop and Toht (796), and their terminology has been followed in the designations listed above. Note the similarities in energy distribution for the "normal" and "pharyngeal" voices, and the random inharmonic energy, that is to say "noise," in the "buccal" voice.

ability of voice. Most important were pitch and pitch variability. High pitch and more variable pitch were either more acceptable than low and monotonous pitch to the listeners, or were correlated with some untested factor which helped to determine acceptability.

It is probably in terms of the general effectiveness of the voice that the artificial larynx is so consistently derogated in the literature. A common theme is the monotonous, mechanical, metallic voice produced by the reed-type instrument. Electronic larynges produced in the 1960's have considerably better timbre. However, the monotony remains in most instruments; in others, the buzz of the carrier frequency may detract from the quality and may mask the speech of the user.

Barney, Haworth, and Dunn (34) have discussed the problem of the quality of the artificial larynx at some length. Their experimentation shows that the introduction of the vocal source into the articulatory system in the pharynx produces a better voice than the same source introduced into the oral cavity. They use this evidence to justify the use of the throat tissue vibration principle in the Western Electric, Type 5,™ electronic larynx. Further comparisons between artificial larynges are needed to establish this point. One thesis, presented by Wallach (798), did confirm that a throat-vibrator artificial larynx, an Aurex Compact,™ was both more intelligible and more "preferred" than a mouth-vibrator, a Cooper-Rand Electrolarynx.™ The Western Electric Type 5,™ however, was not included in the comparison. Greene's (280) report of the clinically established preference for the Aurex Neovox,™ a throat vibrator, has already been mentioned. In a further study by Barney, Haworth, and Dunn (34), a series of comparisons was made between vowels produced by a speaker while using his normal voice and those produced while using an artificial larynx. Certain of the vowels had too much power in the upper harmonics, others too little. The experimenters concluded that the spectrum of the vibrator was, on the average, adequate as a source of harmonics of vowel production.

The implications of these studies to the therapist are important. The observation that the vocal source should be in the lower pharynx, or perhaps below, is a justification for the development of the pseudoglottis at this point. The advantage to the esophageal speaker in being able to make modifications in the way in which he produces the esophageal voice is underlined by the failure of the artificial larynx to produce the harmonic structure of all vowels. In teaching the use of the artificial larynx, one of the major objectives is the adjustment of the articulators to compensate for the limitations of the vocal source.

The evidence is not completely on the side of the esophageal voice. Hyman's (343) study of the esophageal voice and the air-driven reed larynx deals, at one point, with listeners' preferences. In a series of pair comparisons, the artificial-larynx speakers were chosen as "more pleasant to listen to" than the esophageal speakers in every case. It is difficult to reconcile this result to the almost universal condemnation of the quality of the artificial larynx. The writer will not attempt to do so, although in fairness it must be said that such condemnations may logically be based on criteria other than the perception of quality per se. It has been found by McCroskey and Mulligan (490) that the artificial larynx is more intelligible than esophageal speech to the listener who is unfamiliar with esophageal voice. The opposite was true for listeners who had training in speech rehabilitation; these included both speech pathologists and students in training. The latter result was also noted by Shames, Font, and Matthews (678), whose scorers were undergraduate students.

Because of inherent and unavoidable weaknesses in McCroskey and Mulligan's experimental design, generalizations from their results must be tentative. The present writer, however, questions their interpretation of the experimental results. They suggest that professional biases influenced the intelligibility scores. It is difficult to see how biases could affect intelligibility as they measured it. A more tenable hypothesis would be that the naive listener needs to become accustomed to esophageal speech, but may then find it more intelligible than the artificial larynx. If accustomization were demonstrated to be more important for the listener to esophageal voice, the feelings of users of artificial larynges that they were less easily understood, reported by Mc-

Croskey and Mulligan (490), would be shown to be based in fact. It should also be pointed out that most esophageal speakers talk much of the time to listeners who are familiar with their voices. In such circumstances, esophageal speech may be preferred to the artificial larynx because of greater intelligibility. Further study is, of course, indicated.

To summarize the present section, a framework has been established for therapy procedures for the improvement of the quality of esophageal and artificial-larynx speech. To improve quality, an esophageal speaker should concentrate on producing vowels that are open, intelligible, clearly differentiated, and controlled. That is to say, "freely moving" vowels and "smooth" vowels that have full duration in connected speech are basic to quality as well as intensity. Reduction of breathing noises and of struggle with voice production is also of great importance. The user of the artificial larynx, too, needs to learn to compensate for the harmonic defects of his vocal source, and the basic release of the tongue from the laryngeal structures. Thus, vowel practice — similar to that recommended for the esophageal speaker in the sense that open, intelligible, clearly differentiated vowels should be mastered — should be undertaken by the speaker who uses the artificial larynx.

Chapter VIII

Asai Speech: A Special Case of Phonation after Total Laryngectomy and Laryngoplasty

JOHN C. SNIDECOR

Introduction

A NEW TYPE OF total laryngectomy with laryngoplasty is pictured in Figure 3, Chapter I. The process of the operation itself is described and pictured by Dr. Alden Miller in Chapter III. Brief comments are made by this writer (J.C.S.) regarding the nature of Asai speech at the end of Dr. Miller's chapter.

During the fall of 1967, the present writer, with Drs. Nobuhiko Isshiki (Kyoto) and Teru Kimura (Kobe), investigated some of the physiological and acoustical parameters of Asai speech. At that time, approximately one hundred of these laryngoplasty operations had been performed in Japan, most of them at the University of Kobe and a few by Dr. Iwai, a former student of Dr. Asai, at the University of Kyoto Hospital. It was possible to observe the operation as done by Dr. Asai and to study the speech of his patients.

The medical world first gained a complete preview of the operation by means of a detailed motion picture in color presented at the Congress on Cancer, Tokyo, Japan, in October of 1966. The delicate three-stage operation has been highly praised by surgeons in many countries. One famous surgeon called it a "brave" operation. Dr. Asai, after completing the third stage of his operation, stated to this writer that this, the most delicate part of the surgical procedures, was "a minor operation," and in terms of danger to the patient this is true.

The most dramatic example of the Asai operation in the United States was the operation performed on Corporal Walter Lopata which was reported in *Newsweek* of January 23, 1967.

---

*This chapter is based on a report prepared by J. Snidecor, N. Isshiki, and T. Kimura for the XIVth Congress of the International Association of Logopedics and Phoniatrics, September 1968.

Lopata lost his larynx as a result of grenade fragments which tore his larynx away. Dr. William W. Montgomery of the Massachusetts Eye and Ear Infirmary of Boston and Lieutenant Commander Robert Toohill operated on Lopata with the basic Asai operation. They turned the dermal tube downward into the hypopharynx, a procedure discussed by Dr. Miller in Chapter III and utilized currently by Drs. Asai and Iwai. Directing the tube downward limits the entrance of liquids into the tube and has no adverse effect on speech.

The writer has a recording of Lopata's voice shortly after the operation and again four months later. In the first recording, the voice is intelligible but sounds highly artificial and is poorly modulated. In the second recording, a rate of 211 words per minute is maintained; the voice is relatively natural but somewhat hoarse and breathy. (For details regarding voice quality, see Chapter VII.) Modulation is good. No doubt a reduction in rate to something approximating a normal rate of 165 words per minute would reduce the breathiness and improve the overall performance. No pneumographic record was available, but it proved easy to judge when breaths were taken because of breathing noise that was noticeable, but less so than stoma noise in the average esophageal speaker. In a seventy-two-word passage, Lopata used six breaths, or 12 words per breath, a value essentially identical with the average for six normal and superior speakers studied by Snidecor (711).

In the United States, it was not possible as of mid-1967 to find a sufficient number of Asai speakers for more than a very preliminary statement. In Japan, of course, there was no difficulty in selecting subjects. The ones used in this study were supplied by Dr. Kimura of Kobe University.

Selection of Speakers

Five speakers with a wide range of abilities were selected, (3 females and 2 males of middle age). Three judges who were experienced with Asai speech and with esophageal speech rated readings of a fifty-one-word passage read aloud as if to an audience of twenty-five people. The speakers ranged from one to five on a five-point scale on which five is excellent, one is poor, two is fair, three is average, and four is good. There was complete and independent agreement that each speaker fitted one of the five numerical categories. However, even the poorest speaker could use his speech for day-to-day activities. The best speaker, a male, could not be distinguished from a good normal speaker with a slight case of laryngitis.

Procedures

The five Asai speakers performed several special tasks which have been used before to describe esophageal and/or normal speech. Four normal Japanese speakers of matched age and sex performed the same tasks. A fifth normal control failed to complete the assignment and is excluded from these discussions.

The tasks were as follows (see Table I) : (1) The vowel /a/ was phonated as long as possible. (2) The mean flow rate and volume were measured by means of apparatus comparable to that described in Chapter IX, but of Japanese design and manufacture (San'ei) . (3) The intensity level of /a/ was measured as phonated with "comfortable loudness," as were three nonsense syllables. (4) Levels were measured by means of a sound level recorder (Japan Electronics, Ltd.) and recorded by two observers. (5) Frequency for the vowel /a/ was taken from a Japanese-designed "sonagraph." (6) All of the speakers then read a Japanese translation of the "Rainbow Passage" (see Table II) , which in that language proved to have 86 syllables. Syllables per breath, words (U.S.) per breath, syllables per minute, and words per minute (U.S.) were computed as was the ratio of phonated time to total time.

It will be noted that words per breath and words per minute are stated in United States values. These estimates appeared desirable so that data could be compared with those of superior esophageal and superior normal speakers speaking English and previously studied by Snidecor and Isshiki (710) and Snidecor (707) . For those unacquainted with Japanese, these adjustments were desirable because the Japanese compound words and thus use fewer words than are used in English. On the other hand,

TABLE I
SPECIAL TASKS

	Asai Speakers in Order of Preference					Superior Eso.	Japanese Controls				Normal U.S.
	E♂	H♀	O♀	M♂	K♂		A	S	T	W	
Judges' ratings	5	4+	3	2	1+						
Duration [a] (sec)	13.07	4.92	12.00	3.30	3.45	1.16 – 4.25 Berlin 2.8 mean	25.55	22.65	20.30	30.60	12.3 – 59.0
Mean flow cc/sec [a]	350.53	504.90	94.70	143.9	419.40	20–100 (72 M)	106.64	65.61	90.08	52.36	93.7 ♀ 112.4 ♂
Total volume [a] (cc)	4581	2671	1136	475	1441	78–253	2725	1427	1827	1602	
"Comfortable loudness," [a] sustained	75	75	77	80	72	***	78	78	70	70	
"Comfortable loudness," dB for 3 syllables Micro. = 25 cm	67	72	71	74	71	***	73	77	69	67	
Frequency (Hz) [a]	99	214	126	126	126		**	**	**	**	
Counting	25	20	20	13	10	8*	60	50	43	60	40–60*

*Estimate.
**Not available.
***Not available under identical conditions.

TABLE II
PERFORMANCE ON READING PASSAGE (RAINBOW)

	Asai Speakers in Order of Preference					Superior Eso.	Japanese Controls				Normal U.S.
	E♂	H♀	O♀	M♂	K♂		A	S	T	W	
No. breaths 86 syllables	3	5	5	23	12	13.8*	2	12	4	4	5
Syllables/breath	28.66	17.20	17.20	3.74	7.17	5.8*	42	7.17	21.50	21.50	17.5
U.S. words/breath	21.40	12.80	12.80	2.3	5.30	4.2*	31	9.60	15.2	15.2	12.5
Syllables/min	198.36	296.52	132.30	156.36	120.18	135	303.60	156.36	238.80	234.00	189–270
U.S. words/min	147	215	98	116	89	100	224	116	176	173	140–185
Phon. time Total time	.79	.81	.49	.51	.50	.45	.69	.66	.38	.74	.60–.75
Mean Frequency (Hz)	96	150	81	124	80	63		109 – 150♂ 198 – 228♀			132♂ 220♀

*Approximate mean performance, air-charge.

more syllables are used to express the same ideas. The fifty-one-word "Rainbow Passage" in English contains thirty-seven words in Japanese: 66 syllables in English, but 86 syllables in Japanese. In other terms, the Japanese word contained an average of 2.3 syllables per word. The simple expedient of applying the U.S. ratio to the Japanese syllables gives a reasonable estimate of the U. S. words encompassed by one breath and the rate in words per minute in English. Mean frequency levels were estimated from sonagrams. More detailed pitch analysis is planned for a future study. Finally, the subjects counted as high as they felt they could on one breath, a simple task often used for estimates of vocal efficiency.

It should be noted that none of our speakers has had formal speech therapy. Speakers E, H, and O, rated superior to adequate, were in excellent physical condition. Speaker M, rated as a fair speaker, suffered from extensive carcinomatous involvement prior to the operation and gave one the impression of physical weakness. Speaker K, rated as a poor speaker, was in the hospital and ambulatory following his third and final stage of the operation. His stoma at this point appeared rather large, and he had some difficulty in getting a complete closure with thumb or fingers.

Results and Discussion

The results for Special Tasks are summarized in Table I. The duration of the vowel /a/ averages longer for the Asai speakers than for esophageal speakers but substantially shorter than the duration for normal speakers. The high value of 13.07 seconds is about four times that of the esophageal speaker, but only approximately one-half that for the normal speaker.

With the exception of speaker O, mean flow rate far exceeds that of the Japanese and U. S. normal speakers. Flow rate is obviously related to breathiness, so this finding supports that of Nichols stated in Chapter VII on quality and loudness.

With the exception of speaker M, a fair speaker, the total volume of air used is not markedly different from that used by a normal speaker, but all speakers used substantially more air than do esophageal speakers for the same task.

Observing now "Counting" at the bottom of Table I, it will be noted that none of the Asai speakers exceeded any of the normal speakers, but all of them could count higher on one breath than could the average esophageal speakers on one air-charge. W, an exceptional speaker, studied by Snidecor and Isshiki (711), exceeded the count of speakers M (fair) and K (poor). Many of the high counts attributed to superior esophageal speakers are a result of small "plosive backflows" overlaid on larger "inhalations" or tongue pumps, and this phenomenon shows up clearly when subjects are measured by sensitive airflow apparatus.

There is no doubt but that phonatory efficiency in Asai speech falls between the efficiency of normal speech and that for esophageal speech, minor individual differences not to the contrary withstanding.

When comfortable loudness (intensity) of phonation is considered, the trends are surprisingly consistent and in an unexpected direction, that is, the Asai speakers were as loud as the normal speakers. The mean value of 76 dB is the same for both classes of speakers for the phonation /a/. For three syllables of nonsense, *ko ko ni,* the Asai speaker's mean value was 71 dB and the normal speaker's value was 72 dB. Only very superior esophageal speakers match these intensity levels.

Frequency (Hz) values, on the basis of preliminary estimates, show greater differences, although here values for the Japanese controls are not available, but adequate norms from other sources are available. Precise norms are available for male esophageal speakers but not for females. However, in this case, enough general comparisons have been made to make the reasonable assumption that values for male and female esophageal speakers are very close. Here both Table I and Table II require examination in order to note differences between the mean frequency for phonation of /a/ and the mean frequency of the eighty-six-syllable passage. All speakers have a higher frequency for /a/ than for the reading passage as a whole. Because the /a/ was phonated at normal pitch, and because these values at this moment have been more precisely measured, only the phonation of /a/ will be discussed. Although the vowel was higher in pitch than the mean for continuous speech, it probably represents a potential for each speaker. Speaker E (superior male) has a low phonation (99 Hz) for a male voice, falling between that for a normal male speaker (132 Hz) and an esophageal male speaker (63 Hz). Speaker H (good female) has a mean level for /a/ of 214 Hz, essentially the same as the 220 Hz for superior normal female speakers studied by Snidecor (706). Female speaker O (adequate female) phonates at 126 Hz, a value essentially that of the normal male speakers [Pronovost (200)]. Speakers M (fair male) and K (poor male) phonate at 126 Hz, a figure again at the level of the normal male voice.

In general, the speakers had substantially higher voices than values found for esophageal speakers by Damsté (151) and Curry and Snidecor (142). Specific to speaker E, the lowest-pitched speaker, we note that his 99 Hz value is 36 Hz higher than the highest mean level (63 Hz) for six superior esophageal speakers studied by Snidecor and Curry (709). From the level of 63 Hz, the addition of 36 Hz represents half an octave, a substantial difference in perceived pitch level. *Note:* All information on pitch is subject to more definitive analysis.

Temporal values as presented in Table II require speaker-by-speaker analysis. Four out of five of the Asai speakers encompassed more words per breath than superior esophageal speakers did per air-charge. Only speakers M and K (fair and poor speakers respectively), fell substantially below the mean figure of 12 words per breath stated by Snidecor (707) for superior normal readers. E, the best Asai speaker, and A, a Japanese control, spoke 21 and 31 words per breath, proving certainly that the superior Asai speaker can make outstanding use of his air supply.

In terms of words per minute, we find discrepancies in scores which range, for all classes of speakers, from well below averages for normal speakers (i.e. 96, 81, 80, 63, and 116 words per minute) to well above these norm (i.e. 215 and 224 words per minute) for one Asai speaker (good female) and one male Japanese control. Lopata, one of the few American Asai speakers operated on in the United States, exceeded 200 words per minute. The figures between 144 and 185 were established as a normal range of speaking rate by Franke for propositional speech similar to that represented by the passage used in this study. Out of more than one hundred esophageal speakers surveyed by Snidecor, only one fell within this normal range with a rate of 153 words per minute when reading a fifty-one-word prose passage.

Summary

Five Asai speakers, jury rated from one (poor) to five (superior), were studied relative to esophageal and normal speakers. Generally speaking, the Asai speakers fell between the normals and the esophageal speakers for specially assigned tasks and for the reading of a standard propositional prose passage: (1) Duration of the phonation of the vowel /a/ fell between the normal and the esophageal speaker. (2) Airflow rate was high supporting Nichols' judgments in regard to breathy quality. (3) Actual volume of air used was similar to the normal speaker and higher than that used by the esophageal speaker. (4) Counting ability on one breath usually fell between that of normal and esophageals. (5) Normal and Asai speakers demonstrated about the same loudness levels. (6) The Asai speakers were more likely to have pitch levels high and approximating the normal rather than similar to the lower-pitched esophageal speakers. (7) Although not always evidenced, Asai speakers could often speak as many words on one breath as normal speakers, and more words than could the esophageal speakers on one air-charge. (8) Certain Asai speakers far exceeded a desirable rate in words per minute as did one of the Japanese controls. No esophageal speaker yet studied and reported has achieved a rate of speech more rapid than "low normal."

Chapter IX

Airflow in Esophageal Speech

NOBUHIKO ISSHIKI

A IR VOLUME and especially airflow are of great importance in the total act of esophageal speech. Previous studies have, of necessity, been limited in describing such phenomena by the limitations of available spirometric, pneumographic, and radiographic equipment. Nevertheless, previous workers have effectively measured and estimated the temporal and general volumetric aspects of esophageal speech but have not been able to measure the complex and at times minute nature of airflow. The present study was made possible by the development of apparatus recently and specifically designed for airflow studies. Differences in research findings between this and previous studies can be explained in the main by two factors. First, there are many fine movements within the grosser movements which have previously been reported. Second, the speakers in several previous studies have been selected as superior from large groups of speakers. This study analyzed speakers who ranged from adequate to superior. Speakers W and A in this study — speaker W being much better than A — are the only speakers whose performances probably equalled the performances studied, for example, by Kaiser (377), Sugano (747), and Snidecor (710).

Kaiser (377), using a Gad's air volume recorder, studied the aerodynamic aspect of esophageal voice for the first time. She reported that an excellent esophageal speaker insufflated air, generally a little less than 100 cc, before speech. Based on the spirometric or radiographic findings, the volume of air per syllable or per word was reported by Stetson (730), Howie (334), and Snidecor (710). Sugano (747) stated that the air volume expired out of the esophagus ranged from 45 cc to 140 cc. So far as the available literature is concerned, no systematic and analytic measurement of airflow rate or its volume during esophageal speech appears to have been previously reported.

Procedures

Six male esophageal speakers were studied in the present investigation. All of the speakers were intelligible, and even the poorer speakers were judged as belonging in the automatic category described by Wepman *et al.* (807).

The tasks the subjects performed included reading a part of the "Rainbow Passage," sustaining phonations of the vowel /a/, counting as high as possible with one breath, articulating CVC syllables, swallowing, and breathing.

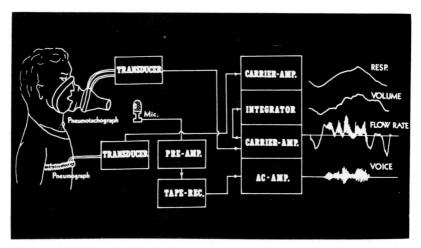

FIGURE 34. Diagram of the experimental arrangement.

An outline of the experimental arrangement is illustrated in Figure 34. Four measurements were made simultaneously during esophageal speech: (1) the voice, (2) the respiratory (thoracic) movement, (3) rate, and (4) volume of airflow through the oronasal passage. The subjects wore air-tight masks during speech so that no air could leak between the face and mask. Voice signals were recorded on a tape recorder through a condenser microphone. The output of the tape recorder was, in turn, connected via an AC amplifier to a four-channel polybeam recorder to obtain an oscillographic recording of voice. The movement of the thorax was recorded by means of a pneumograph. A pressure variation in the pneumograph was sensitized by a strain gauge pressure transducer and recorded on another channel of the recorder.

A pneumotachograph was utilized to measure the rate of airflow in and out of the mouth and nose during speech. Electrical signals from the differential pressure transducer were amplified by a carrier amplifier and fed into one of the four channels of the polybeam recorder so that a tracing of the flow rate was secured. An integrating amplifier converted the flow rate signal into the volume automatically. The pneumotachograph was calibrated by frequent checks with a rotameter. An example of the recordings is shown in Figure 35.

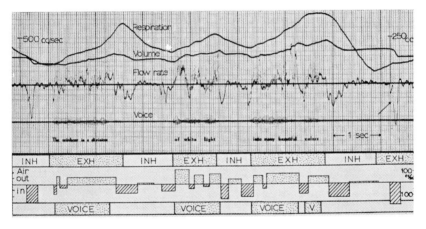

FIGURE 35. From top to bottom the traces represent (1) Respiration. Inhalation is represented by the downward slope, exhalation by the upward curve. (2) Volume of air intake and exsufflation (each heavy graduation, consisting of 5 fine graduations, corresponds to 25 cc). Inward airflow is represented by the downward slope, outward flow by the upward slope. (3) Airflow rate traces above the baseline represent outward flow, below the line inward flow. Each heavy graduation corresponds to 50 cc per sec. (4) Voice. These recordings are schematically shown below by block diagrams. In the second row of the diagram, flow rate is represented by the height of the block, volume by the area. The arrow indicates an asynchronous air intake.

Analyses of Recordings

In analyzing the complicated sequence of events during esophageal speech, three parameters were taken into consideration, as schematically indicated in Figure 34. These were respiratory movement, direction of airflow, and voicing. According to all possible combinations of these three factors, the events during esophageal speech were classified into eight different categories, as shown in Table I. For each type of different event, analyses were made as to the volume and rate of airflow and the duration of the event. In interpreting the data for the airflow, special care was taken so that the flow measured by the pneumotachograph did not directly indicate the airflow into the esophagus. Some movement of air sensitized by the pneumotachograph simply resulted from the slight change in the oropharyngeal cavity because of the tongue movement. In general, it was noted that if the incoming and outgoing flow of air was limited within the cavity above the pseudoglottis, the inward flow of air was immediately followed by the same amount of outward flow of air. On the other hand, all the outgoing airflow accompanied by voice was judged as emanating from the esophagus or from below the pseudoglottis.

TABLE I

Type	Direction of Oronasal Airflow	Phase Relation Between Tracheal and Oronasal Airflow	Voicing or Not	Remarks
1	In	Out-phase	No	Indicative of injection of air
2	In	Out-phase	Voice	
3	In	In-phase	No	Indicative of inhalatory intake
4	In	In-phase	Voice	Inhalatory phonation
5	Out	Out-phase	No	Loss of air or voiceless consonant
6	Out	Out-phase	Voice	Asynchronous phonation
7	Out	In-phase	No	Loss of air or voiceless consonant
8	Out	In-phase	Voice	Synchronous phonation similar to normal

Air Intake

The total amount of air intake while reading the "Rainbow Passage" was about 1000 cc for each of the present subjects, except for the poorest speaker who took in only 325 cc.

TABLE II*
AIR INTAKE

Ranking Subject	1 W	2 A	2 V	3 C	3 M	4 P
Total volume of air intake in cc	948	1118	888	987	1189	325
Total speech time in sec	28	23	29	36	45	29
Rate of air intake in cc/sec	33.9	48.6	30.6	27.4	26.4	11.2
Synchronous intake of air (during inhalation) in vol %	76	9	62	64	71	44
Asynchronous intake of air (during exhallation)	24	91	38	36	29	56
Synchronous intake of air (during inhalation) in time percentage	66	16	48	49	64	43
Asynchronous intake of air (during exhalation)	34	84	52	51	36	57
Voiced air intake in vol %	14	67	35	21	21	45
Unvoiced air intake in vol %	86	33	65	79	79	55
No. of respirations	14	3	24	26	36	25

*The data were obtained from recording the airflow during the reading of the "Rainbow Passage."

If the efficiency of air intake is judged by the rate of air intake per unit of time (total air intake per total speech time including the pause between speech), it is noted that the better the speakers, the more efficient the air intake.

Phase Relationship Between Air Intake and Respiration

The inhalation method implies, by definition, that the intake of air is synchronous with the inhalatory movement of the thorax; in the injection method, the intake of air can take place during exhalation as well as inhalation. If the air is insufflated during exhalation or asynchronously with the breathing, it appears that the air was taken in by a variation of the injection method, not by the inhalation method. Therefore, an analysis of the phase relationship between the intake of air and respiration is helpful in judging the method of air intake which the esophageal speaker is utilizing.

For each of the six subjects, the percentages of air volume insufflated synchronously with the respiration (types 3 and 4 in Table I) during the reading of the "Rainbow Passage" are shown in Table II and in Figure 36. Most speakers employ both synchronic and asynchronic intake of air in various degrees, depending on the method of air intake. The majority of speakers (inhalation and injection) charged more air synchronously than asynchronously. Speaker A obtained most (91%) of his air during the exhalatory phase. This asynchrony between air intake and respiration indicates that he is principally an injector.

Air Intake With or Without Voicing

If the air is suctioned into the esophagus through the pseudoglottis which is actively opened, the incoming stream of air would not produce voice. If the glottis is closed, air intake may accompany the voicing. If the air is actively injected under a positive pressure through the closed glottis, the airflow is more likely to cause vocalization. From these concepts, the air intake in relation to vocalization is meaningful.

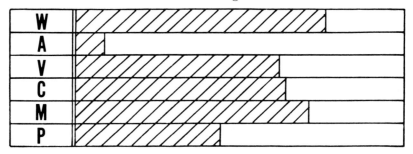

FIGURE 36. Phase relationship between air intake and respiration, expressed in volume percentage. The slashed area represents the air intake during inhalation (synchronous intake), the blank area the air intake during exhalation (asynchronous intake).

The volume ratio of air insufflation with voice (types 2 and 4 in Table I) to that without voice (types 1 and 3) indicates a great individual variation as shown in Table II and Figure 37. Subject

A (injector) was unique in that a greater volume of air was taken with voicing than without voicing. The other subjects insufflated more air without vocalization than with vocalization. It appears that the voiced air intake occurs mostly during the exhalatory phase (voiced injection method) and very seldom during the inhalatory phase (inhalatory phonation).

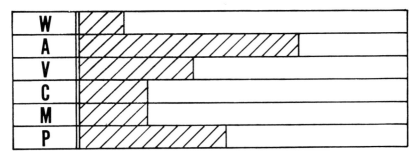

FIGURE 37. Relationship between air intake and voice production. The slashed area represents the voiced air intake, the blank area the voiceless air intake.

Comparison of Four Types of Air Intake

When the two factors of vocalization and the phase relationship with breathing are taken into consideration, the intake of air can be classified into four types as shown in Table I. For all the subjects, the volume of air insufflated by one event of method 3 (in-phase, unvoiced) is greater than that obtained by the other methods (Table III). The intake of air by type 4 (synchronous with respiration, voiced), which represents the inhalatory phonation, is almost negligible. A greater resistance to the incoming airflow is expected when the air intake is accompanied by voice, since during phonation the pseudoglottis is assumed to be closed. This greater resistance of the pseudoglottis to the airflow during phonation may explain why more air can be insufflated without vocalization than with vocalization. So far as the amount of air intake is concerned, method 3 (indicative of the inhalatory method) is most effective. But, method 2 (indicative of the injection method) can be more efficient if the voice produced during the air intake is well articulated and intelligible.

TABLE III
MEAN VOLUME (cc) OF AIR INTAKE DURING ONE EVENT OF
FOUR DIFFERENT METHODS

Method	W	A	Subject V	C	M	P	Mean
Type 1	14.1	11.0	10.0	11.8	9.1	7.0	10.55
Type 2	5.9	13.4	8.1	7.8	6.9	5.4	7.92
Type 3	29.9	17.0	17.0	18.5	21.7	9.9	19.0
Type 4	10.0		10.8		5.7	4.0	7.62

TABLE IV
MEAN DURATION (SEC) OF AIR INTAKE DURING ONE EVENT
OF FOUR DIFFERENT METHODS

Method	W	A	Subject V	C	M	P	Mean
Type 1	.23	.12	.12	.18	.20	.12	.16
Type 2	.12	.11	.11	.17	.13	.16	.13
Type 3	.32	.30	.13	.20	.30	.25	.25
Type 4	.25		.09		.07	.13	.14

One event of air intake by method 3 takes a longer period of time than the other methods (Table IV). If we regard methods 1 and 2 as the injection methods and method 3 as the inhalation method, then the difference in duration of one action between the injection method (types 1 and 2) and the inhalation method (type 3) is quite conceivable because, in general, the duration of the tongue movement appears shorter than that of the breathing movement.

TABLE V
MEAN FLOW RATE (cc/sec) OF AIR INTAKE FOR FOUR
DIFFERENT METHODS

Method	W	A	Subject V	C	M	P	Mean
Type 1	62	96	83	64	46	57	68
Type 2	50	118	71	45	56	33	62
Type 3	94	58	135	95	73	39	82
Type 4	40		123		77	30	70

The flow rates for the different types of air intake are shown in Table V. It is seen that in subject W, V, C, and M, who appeared to utilize primarily the inhalation method, the flow rate for method 3 (indicative of inhalation method) is higher than the flow rate for method 1 or 2 (indicative of the injection method). In contrast, the flow rate for method 1 or 2 (injection) was higher than the flow rate for method 3 (inhalation) for speaker A and P (principally injectors).

Generally, during one inhalatory movement, one or two substantial intakes of air occurred. The better speakers such as W and V were inclined to perform a greater number of air intakes — sometimes three — during one inhalatory phase, as indicated in Figure 35. As observed in 1967, after three years of experience, W consistently charges three times before a loud brief phrase.

Airflow During Swallowing

The swallowing method was not efficient in air-charging. An inward flow of air (usually less than 50 cc) during the initial stage of swallowing was followed by an outward flow of air during the latter stage of swallowing, This phenomenon appears to occur because most of the air movement is limited within the cavity above the pseudoglottis and a very small amount of air may be drawn inefficiently into the esophagus by swallowing. Moreover, the swallowing movement could not be repeated rapidly. Shipp (684) has shown by electromyography that swallowing and injecting are two different neuromuscular acts.

Airflow During Breathing

A normal inhalation itself (not so quick as during speech) did not introduce any inward movement of air through the nose or mouth in any subjects.

Outward Flow of Air

Most of the outward flow of air from the esophagus or oropharyngeal cavity occurred during the exhalatory phase of respiration (synchrony), regardless of the method of air intake (Table VI). A plosive-injector expels a greater amount of air without voice (unmodulated airflow) than with voice (modulated airflow). In the other speakers, most of the outflow of air expelled during the exhalatory phase was used for voice production. Unmodulated airflow does not necessarily mean the loss of air, because it may be contributing to the pronunciation of the voiceless consonants.

TABLE VI
OUTWARD FLOW OF AIR: RELATIONSHIP WITH RESPIRATION
AND VOCALIZATION (Vol %)

	W	A	V	C	M	P
Synchronous outflow (during exhalation)	91	97	85	69	92	77
Asynchronous outflow (during inhalation)	9	3	15	31	8	23
Voiced outflow	83	44	74	50	81	59
Unvoiced outflow	17	56	26	50	19	41

TABLE VII
PHONATION: RELATIONSHIP WITH THE DIRECTION OF
AIRFLOW AND RESPIRATORY PHASE (Vol %)

			Subject			
Method	W	A	V	C	M	P
Type 8	84	40	61	65	73	58
Type 2	13	60	24	32	21	36
Types 4 & 6	3	0	15	3	6	6

Phonation

According to the direction of airflow and the phase relation with respiration, voice production can be classified into four types: (1) using the inward flow during exhalation (asynchronic); (2) using the inward flow during inhalation (synchronic); (3) using the outward flow during inhalation (asynchronic); (4) using the outward flow during exhalation (synchronic). These four different kinds of phonations correspond to the types 2, 4, 6, and 8 respectively in the classification in Table I.

TABLE VIII
THE MEAN FLOW RATES (cc/sec) FOR TWO MAIN TYPES OF
PHONATIONS DURING SPEECH

			Subject				
Method	W	A	V	C	M	P	*Normal*
Type 8	69	97	56	46	66	25	219
Type 2	50	118	71	45	56	33	

In all of the subjects, except A (the plosive-injector), the voice was produced predominantly with the outward flow of air during exhalation (type 8) and, to a lesser degree, produced with the inward flow of air during the exhalatory phase (type 2) (Table VII and Fig. 38). Speaker A produced voice more by utilizing the inward flow during exhalation than by utilizing the outward flow during exhalation.

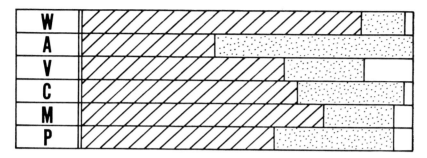

FIGURE 38. Three different types of phonation. The slashed area represents a phonation with outward airflow during exhalation (type 8); the dotted area, a phonation with inward flow of air during exhalation (type 2); the blank area, a phonation during inhalation (types 4 and 6).

The inhalatory phonation (using inflow during the inhalatory phase) was very rare for all the speakers: the volume percentage of the inhalatory phonation to the total phonation ranged from 0 to 8. The mean flow rate during phonation using outward flow of air during exhalation (type 8) ranged from 25 to 97 cc per sec. The mean flow rate for the poorest speaker (P) is substantially lower as compared with those for the other and better speakers. The plosive-injector A uses a very high rate of airflow for phonation. All of the foregoing data were obtained from recording the airflow during the reading of the "Rainbow Passage."

The mean flow rates for sustained phonation of the vowel /a/ ranged from 27 to 72 cc per sec. Speaker W continued phonation for a maximum of 4.25 sec. The injectors, A and P, could not prolong the vowel /a/ as long as the other speaker could. The difference in the flow rates between voiceless consonants and voiced consonants was not as distinct in esophageal speech as in normal speech.

Injector and Inhaler

It was revealed that the types of air intake and usage in connection with respiration and vocalization vary greatly with the speakers. Furthermore, it was suggested that most of the esophageal speakers used a combination of methods of air intake. In order to contrast the differences among those methods, a comparison is made between speakers W and A, both of whom were superior in esophageal speech and were considered as representing the two different types of esophageal speech.

Speaker W took most of the air (76%) during inhalatory phase of respiration (synchronous intake), while speaker A pumped in almost all the air (91%) during the exhalatory phase (asynchronous intake). A similar tendency was found in time percentage of air intake. In speaker W, only 14 per cent of the total volume of air intake was accompanied by voice. In speaker A, 67 per cent of the total air intake was voiced. Speaker W breathed fourteen times while reading the fifty-one-word passage, but A breathed only three times during the same passage; a normal subject took six breaths for the same passage.

In speaker A, the expiration occurred very gradually and slowly. The noise level produced by both speakers at the tracheostoma was too low to attract any attention. The speeches by the two subjects were equally intelligible. A's speech, however, was characterized by his overaccentuation of plosive consonant sounds. In the performance of prolonged phonation of the vowel /a/, speaker W was much superior to speaker A in that W sustained the vowel /a/ much longer than did A. Speaker W repeated syllable /ma/ air in connection with the plosive consonant (see Fig. 39).

A synchronous intake of air (air intake during inhalation) alone, although highly indicative of the inhaler, is not sufficient to conclude that one is purely an inhaler, because the injection of air

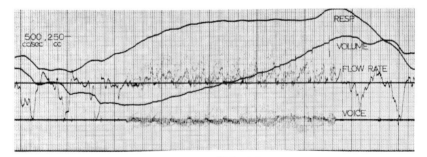

FIGURE 39. Maximum repetition (14 times) of the syllable /ba/ with one breath by speaker W. Note that no air intake occurred in connection with the syllable /ba/.

can occur theoretically during the inhalatory phase too. The question is whether or not the speaker is using the tongue to pump air. The recording of airflow showed that the normal deep (not so quick as during speech) breathing movement itself, without any movement of the tongue, did not induce any substantial inflow of air through the oronasal passage.

Some portion of air was taken in also during exhalation (asynchronous intake) as indicated by the arrow in Figure 35. The two separate intakes of air during one inhalatory phase, as shown in the same Figure, appeared to correspond to two movements of the tongue. Furthermore, to an inquiry about his method of air intake, speaker W answered that he could not charge air without the movement of the tongue. From these findings, it was assumed that W was also using the tongue-pumping method (injection). From reasoning similar to the above, the other subjects were also considered as using both inhalation and injection methods, although the degree of dominance of one method over the other appeared to vary with the speakers.

Advantages and Disadvantages of Various Methods

Naturally, insufflation of air into the esophagus by the tongue movement would be greatly facilitated by negative pressure in the esophagus. Actually one of the advantages of the inhalation method is a large amount of air intake per trial, which can be demonstrated by a sustained phonation of the vowel /a/. As previously mentioned, the mean volume of synchronous intake of air (during inhalation) is greater than the volume insufflated during the exhalatory phase (Table III).

However, it should be mentioned that overexertion of the respiratory movement may result in various disadvantages which have been pointed out by many writers. These include parasitic noise at the tracheostoma, unfavorable effect on the lungs and vascular system, fatigue, and so on. The speakers who repeat deep breathing too frequently during speech, with a great tracheal noise, should be taught more about the use of the tongue and lips in charging air in, and relaxation of, the pseudoglottis as a means of compensation for respiratory overexertion. Too much dependence on the inhalation method may sometimes lead to the difficulties mentioned above. However, these difficulties or disadvantages do not lead to a refutation of the inhalation method at all. The important aspect is the balance of the respiratory effort.

The suppression of the respiratory movement alone does not seem to solve the problem, because this will result in the reduction of the volume of air intake and in the decreased force of air expulsion during phonation. If those noise-producing speakers learned to relax the pseudoglottis or learned the other method of air intake — tongue pumping — the respiratory exertion would naturally be reduced. No further need exists for respiratory over-exertion.

Some movements of the tongue and the other articulatory organs which are used in normal speech before laryngectomy are similar to the movements necessary for air insufflation and therefore can be utilized as cues to the new movements to be learned. These are, for instance, pronunciation of the plosive consonants and swallowing. Many investigators (van Gilse 1949; van den Berg, Moolenaar-Bijl and Damsté 1958; Schlosshauer and Möckel, 1958) have already described the initial phase of swallowing as resembling the action of the tongue required for air insufflation. It should be emphasized to the patient that the total action of swallowing is not appropriate for air intake but only the initial stage need be used.

Earlier work in this area appears to support one particular method and to refute the other methods. Moreover, some of the articles, although they support the various methods, give the impression that the speaker has to choose and use only one method: the methods appeared incompatible with each other. Within the limitation of the present data, we feel that many esophageal speakers are unconsciously employing a combination of methods of air intake, which we think is recommendable.

Chapter X

How Effective Can an Esophageal Speaker Be?

John C. Snidecor

THE QUESTION of the ultimate efficiency of esophageal speech often enters the mind of both teacher and client. To answer this question in part, M. W., a truly superior speaker, was studied in detail. First, his speech is excellent — rapid, clear, and loud enough to be heard in a noisy restaurant or airplane. Second, M. W. is capable of using more air than any other esophageal speaker we have studied experimentally or read or heard about.

> Our speaker is fifty-two years of age, approximately six feet tall, slim, wiry, and physically strong. He is a successful, active person who as an avocation operates single or multi-engined planes. He speaks to crew and control tower. M.W. is generous and outgoing, giving unlimited time to our studies, and apparently enjoying our company as much as we enjoyed his. In brief, he was of an age, and had those physical and personal characteristics described by Schall (639) and Stoll (738) as conducive to the development of effective esophageal speech. M.W. had his operation on April 10, 1963 at the Mayo Clinic, exactly one year before the experiment. He had started to speak ten days after the operation, and twelve days after surgery received his only formal speech therapy, consisting of one long session with Frederic L. Darley, Ph.D. of the Mayo Clinic. Here it should be recalled that many esophageal speakers continue to improve for a period of from three to four years and so it is quite possible that M.W. will improve beyond his current excellence.

The speaker was assigned a variety of vocal tasks which included reading aloud a seventy-syllable "normal" reading passage, counting, prolongation of vowels under various conditions of pitch and loudness, singing the scale, articulated CVC paradigms, and the repetition of various syllabic combinations. Airflow measurements were based on simultaneous recordings of flow rate, air volume, thoracic movement, and voice signals.

The results of this study clearly delineate M. W. as a superior esophageal speaker.

Rate and Duration

One of the best measures of efficiency in speech is rate in words per minute. Darley (200) established rate norms of normal speakers for a passage very similar to the one used here. His zero percentile was represented by 129 words per minute, the fiftieth percentile by 166 words per minute, and the one-hundredth percentile by 222 words per minute. Of especial importance to this study is the Franke (217) investigation of judgment of rate which determined that critical listeners judge rate too rapid if it exceeds 185 words per minute and too slow if it is less than 140 words per minute. A previous study of rate in superior esophageal speech by Snidecor (707) indicated a range of from 108 to 137 words per minute with a median rate of 122.5. Thus no speaker in this earlier study exceeded Darley's fifth percentile, and no speaker would be judged as adequately rapid by the Franke norms.

M. W. is exceptionally rapid for an esophageal speaker. One feels no impatience in listening to his flow of speech. His rate of 153 words per minute is at Darley's fifteenth percentile for normal speakers and within the limits of satisfactory rate for normal speakers as defined by Franke. No other effective esophageal speaker in this study or the Snidecor study is closely competitive (see Table I, columns A, C, M, P, V as regards performance in rate). It is of incidental interest that M. W. can speak even more rapidly, but vocal quality deteriorates with increased rate. The ratio of phonated time to total time gives some measure of vocal efficiency. If the speaker has many and/or long pauses, his effective total rate will be reduced. Moreover, his speech will be either unduly staccato or hesitant, thus distracting from the meaning of his speech. According to Black (78), Hanley (304), and Snidecor (706), normal speakers phonate from 60 to 75 per cent of the time during continuous speech. Table I, item 3, indicates a range of phonated time from 38.4 per cent to 57.4 per cent for esophageal speakers, a figure obviously well below that of approximately .68 for normal speakers. The poor esophageal speaker has badly broken rhythm and is hesitant, whereas the effective esophageal speaker is rhythmical but more staccato than the normal speaker. The ability to count is frequently used as a measure of vocal efficiency for the esophageal speaker, but this proves little since the speaker may take many air-charges if he is an "inhaler." M. W. is an inhaler and can count to fourteen (19 syllables) on one air-charge. He does so in 6.26 seconds, and uses 615 cc of air at a rate of 98 cc per sec. This phenomenal performance is accomplished on one single outflow of air without any directional reversals.

TABLE I
GENERAL TEMPORAL RELATIONSHIPS
Esophageal Speakers

	1* M.W.	2 A	3 C	3 M	4 P	2 V	Normal Speaker
1. Words/min	153	128	80	122	96	122	140–185
2. Syllables/min	210	183	117	168	147	168	203–265
3 Ratio of phonated to total time (%)	50.8	47.0	39.5	38.4	44.0	57.4	60–75
4. Count with one air-charge or breath	14	na†	na	na	na	na	40 est.
5. Duration of /a/ range (sec)	1.16– 4.25	na	na	na	na	na	12.3–59.0
6. Duration of /a/ mean of 10–12 trials (sec)	3.70	na	na	na	na	na	25.7
7. Repetition of /ba/	14						70 est.
8. Repetition of /ma/	15						70 est.

*This and other following numerals on the horizontal represent the average rating of the esophageal speakers.
†Not available.

Intensity Variations

M. W. was able to produce the vowel /a/ instantaneously at the maximum level of 85 dB. A normal speaker can sustain the vowel /a/ at the level of 95 dB. The crescendo-diminuendo exercise is a simple way to check the extent and nature of uninterrupted changes in intensity increases and decreases. A normal speaker, unskilled in singing, averaged smooth intensity changes from low to high (crescendo) and high to low (diminuendo) from 35 to 45 dB. Our superior esophageal speaker averaged about 20 dB for both the upward and downward intensity sweep. Van den Berg, Moolenaar-Bijl, and Damsté (63) report the same value. The intensity increases and decreases for the esophageal speakers are "rough." Nichols (Chapter VII) has shown this on intensity profiles on broad-band sonagrams, and our comparable data agree with his. Both types of speakers had rather abrupt crescendos and more gradual diminuendos.

M. W., in common with other esophageal speakers, has a restricted dynamic range as noted from the crescendo-diminuendo series, and a similar tendency was noted in separate phonations of soft and loud vowels. From the above information, we can see that potential intensity levels and variability are much less for the esophageal speaker than the normal speaker. The efficiency of the sound-producing system, though suprisingly effective, is less effective than for the normal speaker. The intensity-modulating system is also less sensitive. However, one must hasten to add that when continuous propositional speech is under consideration, sound pressure levels and variability are essentially the same for each speaker. In fifty-one words of propositional speech, on the basis of measuring peak values, this esophageal speaker has a mean value of 77 dB, the normal speaker of 79 dB. The method of peak measurement may slightly exaggerate values in continuous speech, but the relative values are stable and dependable.

Pitch Level and Flexibility

The pitch of the effective male esophageal speaker is substantially lower than the pitch of the normal male voice. Both the Damsté (151) data and Curry-Snidecor (142) data reveal that mean frequency levels are about one octave below those for normal speakers. The Curry-Snidecor data gave detailed consideration to pitch variability and noted that superior esophageal speakers have a speaking range from 2.0 to 2.5 octaves with an SD in tones of 2.30. This variability in pitch is comparable to that of the normal speaker, as reported by Pronovost (200). However, the human perceptual mechanism does not appreciate the actual variability in Hz. Stevens and Volkmann (734) present experimental data which clearly indicate that in the frequency region below 100 Hz the perceptual or pitch aspects of a stimulus are greatly reduced when compared with frequencies about 100 Hz.

Pitch and Intensity

The relation between pitch and intensity is complicated. It appears, in general, that the increase in intensity is accompanied by the increase in pitch and vice versa. This tendency is especially distinct during the time that the pitch or intensity is varied continuously during one phonation such as crescendo, diminuendo, or singing scale. However, a very high-pitched voice could be produced with relatively low intensity, particularly when M. W. attempted to produce a high-pitched voice with a small amount of air left in the esophagus or stomach at the end of phonation. Occasionally, he could also produce a low loud voice, but it was rather difficult for him to repeat this performance. In other words, the vocal pitch and intensity could be changed intentionally to some extent, but it is not very percisely controlled. These findings are in general agreement with the findings by van den Berg and Moolenaar-Bijl (62) and suggest that M. W. has a slight control of the pseudoglottis probably through the cricopharyngeal muscle and its simple innervation.

Vocal Quality

In reference to quality or wave-form information, spectrographic analysis of esophageal voice revealed that although the voice contains a noise component up to a high-frequency region (6,000 Hz), the harmonic components are still clear and easily distinguishable from each other. When the voice is high in pitch, the noise component is relatively great, and the pitch is unstable as noted in irregular "vertical striations" of a wide-band sonagram. Such a high-pitched voice is usually produced with great strain. A narrow-band sonagram shows the general tendency that an increase in intensity is accompanied by a relative accentuation of high-frequency components.

Mean Flow Rate

M. W.'s mean flow rate during the longest phonation of /a/ ranged from 20 to 75 cc per sec for soft or medium voice and from 85 to 100 cc per sec for loud voice. (Mean flow rate for his easy phonation was 72 cc per sec.) As to the flow rate in normal adults, Isshiki and von Leden (357) found that it ranges from about 70 to 180 cc per sec for most comfortable sustained phonation of the vowel /a/. The range of flow rate for extreme phonation (upper and lower limits in pitch and intensity) is naturally wider, from about 40 to 360 cc per sec. The flow rate for loud and high-pitched voice is greater in general than for soft and low-pitched voice. There appears to be no previous report with respect to the flow rate in esophageal speech, except that by van der Berg, Boolenaar-Bijl and Damsté (63), who deduced that mean flow rate as about 40 cc per sec from spirometric measurement of air intake and maximum phonation time. The mean flow rate of phonation /a/ for the other six esophageal speakers tested at our laboratory ranged from 27 to 49 cc per sec, while the corresponding value for M. W. was 72 cc per sec. From these data, it may well be concluded that the M. W.'s flow rate for continuous phonation /a/ is located around the lower limit of range for normal subjects but considerably higher than for the other esophageal speakers.

Air Reservoir

The maximum capacity of the esophagus and/or stomach as an air reservoir has been of great interest and controversy in esophageal speech. Voorhoeve (790) observed roentgenographically that the stomach contains the air during speech. Beck (47) stated that the stomach is not used as an air reservoir in trained speakers but only occasionally in beginners. Van den Berg and Moolenaar-Bijl wrote that they had never seen an esophageal speaker who fills the stomach with air. In M. W., the total air volume expelled continuously from the mouth and nose, without any directional reversals, was measured ten times while he sustained the vowel /a/ as long as he could. It ranged from 78 to 253 cc. These values were surprisingly great, as compared with those for the other esophageal speakers tested (mostly below 50 cc). However, to our further surprise, once when he attempted to count as far as he could (from 1 to 14) with one breath, the amount of air expelled during that period (6.26 sec) reached the value of 615 cc. The rate of flow was 98 cc per sec. Obviously, these values of total amount of air depend partly on the actual capacity of air-containable organs and partly on how deeply or how many times he charged the air in, without eructation.

The capacity of the esophagus was evaluated as about 80 cc by van den Berg and Moolenaar-Bijl (60) . From these data, it seems obvious that M. W. is using or can use the stomach as an air reservoir. As a matter of fact, he told us he had a cushion of air in the stomach. This was difficult for us to believe until the airflow was actually measured. Figure 39 is a sample of the superior speaker's performance. The caption explains the nature of the performance.

Our superior speaker (W) used as much air and sometimes even more air than a superior speaker carefully studied and described by Kaiser (377) . Both Kaiser's speaker and M. W. use the stomach as a reservoir for air. Air in excess of 80 cc must be so stored. Both speakers were aware of an air cushion, and Voorhoeve's x-rays (presented by Kaiser) give clear evidence of a substantial air bubble that diminishes during speech. Speaker W, with a maximum air-charge of over 600 cc, obviously has a large gastric bubble.

However, attention should be directed to the fact that this enormous amount of air is not usually utilized during conversation or reading. It simply indicates the possibility of his skill.

Relation Between Phonation and Respiration

In earlier times, many authors such as Schilling (640) and Kallen (380) observed or further recommended dissociation or discoordination between phonation and respiration in esophageal speech. On the other hand, more recent investigators seem to be in agreement as to synchrony between these two phenomena. Stetson (730) supported synchronism on the basis of spirometric findings. Snidecor and Curry (709) , using an electropneumograph and phonophotographic equipment, indicated a synchronous tendency between phonation and respiration. A study by Robe *et al.* (622) , through the use of a graphic recording apparatus and motion picture, further presented data which were in favor of synchrony between oral and pulmonary air movements. M. W. produced voice 97 per cent of the time on the exhalatory phase.

M. W. has been observed regularly since April of 1964. His speech has improved in loudness but otherwise appears unchanged. Air intake, once with some dominance on "inhalation," is now dominantly by injection.

Chapter XI

The Charging and Expulsion of Esophageal Air

JOHN C. SNIDECOR

THE FUNDAMENTAL act in learning esophageal speech is the charging and releasing of air from the esophagus, and the most difficult aspect of this two-sided problem for most patients is that of getting air into the esophagus.

There are three well-established methods of charging air described briefly by Travis (777) and others. The author believes that these, or at least two of the methods, are normally used in combination — frequently without consciousness on the part of the speaker. Although the proponents of each "system" wax enthusiastic over their methodology, and often condemn others, the present writer believes in the validity of all three methods and would exclude none of them. This view has recent support in a study by Isshiki and Snidecor (356) and by studies of a very superior speaker by Snidecor and Isshiki (711). It will be noted that each of the three methods discussed below is supported by those with clinical experience, and each method appears to be supported by at least one competent roentgenological study.

I. The Suction, "Breathing," or Inhalation Method

This method is strongly supported by the radiological studies of Hodson and Oswald (325) in England, and is described in their brief but excellent monograph entitled *Speech Recovery After Total Laryngectomy*. Seeman (666), of Prague, a very experienced and highly successful therapist, insists on inhalation in much the same manner described by Hodson and Oswald. He is very insistent that swallowing movements are uneconomical and should be avoided.

In the Hodson and Oswald x-ray studies, air was seen to enter the top of the esophagus accompanied by a rapid downward movement of the diaphragm. The diaphragm served as the chief muscle of "inspiration" and in no case with skilled speakers did the air enter the stomach. No movement of the swallowing mechanism was observed, although there was a slight movement of the neck and chin which might initially be confused with a swallowing movement.

At first, Hodson and Oswald have their patients informally associate with esophageal speakers and listen only. Some speech usually develops as a result, in large part, of listening. Later, after some progress has been made, the patient is taught to "breathe" with the diaphragm, blow mouth organs, whistle, and hum. Obviously, in the case of the mouth organs and whistling, the glossopharyngeal press is brought into action.

Air is released "largely by diaphragmatic action" through a narrowed segment at the top of the esophagus which vibrates, thus serving as the basis for voice. Along with the movement of the diaphragm, one observes a narrowing of the esophagus from below, which may indicate a true muscular or "antiperistaltic" movement. "Certainly the main expulsive force seems to be the act of expiration."

The writer would attempt to describe the feel of charging air by this method by stating that the individual should imagine that he has gas to the point of discomfort in the top of the gullet and desires to release it. The top of the esophagus is relaxed and the diaphragm pulled sharply downward, which usually causes air to be taken into the esophagus, and the air and any gas present will be released at once, normally with a belching sound. As the patient learns to charge and release air with skill, he "breathes" into the top of the esophagus and releases the air at will with appropriate vibration in the cricopharyngeal region.

The cricopharyngeal region is the usual vibrator, but Diedrich (172) points out there are five possible sites for the approximation of tissue in the pharyngo-esophageal vestibule: (1) the superior esophageal sphincter, (2) the cricopharyngeal muscle, (3) the inferior pharyngeal constrictor in opposition to the anterior pharyngeal constrictor, (4) the middle constrictor forming transverse mucosal folds, and (5) the lingual pharyngeal approximation. In a later study, Diedrich and Youngstrom (174) locate the P-E segment in terms of the vertebra at which it operates most of the time. On the basis of meticulous x-ray studies, they found that the level of the segment ranges from C_3 to C_7 with C_5, C_{5-6}, and C_6 being the most common location.

Esophageal speakers taught by the "suction" or "breathing" method can become very effective. This method is taught by many British therapists, and the writer has heard good speakers who use this method. However, Fontaine and Mitchell (214) of Oxford generally use injection methods.

In the United States, therapists are inclined to be eclectic; so some speakers are taught to inhale and, generally speaking, the results are satisfactory.

II. Air Injection by Tongue and Related Structures

The tongue-injection method can be used to produce effective, clear speech. It is endorsed by such expert esophageal speakers and teachers as Nelson (538) in his booklet *You Can Speak Again,* and by Doehler (176) in her pamphlet *Esophageal Speech.* The instructional recording by Doehler, of course, recommends this method. Hyman's recent training recording suggests this method as acceptable, as do Waldrop and Gould in their recent training manual *Your New Voice.*

Schlosshauer and Möckel (643), using synchronized roentgen sound film for twenty-five subjects, give clear-cut support of the validity of the tongue-injection method. Patient Five, one of their effective speakers, "raises the dorsal surface of the tongue and literally rocks the air from the oral cavity into the pharynx by means of a reversed undulatory motion."

Basically, the air is pumped into the top of the esophagus by a rapid "swallow-like" motion of the tongue. The term "swallow" should never be used even early in instruction. Recent research by Shipp *et al.* (685), using electromyographic methods, indicates clearly that the nature of muscle action in swallowing and air injection is different. The concept of the tongue as a pump was early recognized by the Germans in the use of the term *pump-werke.* The action is one rapid motion with the high point of the tongue acting very much like the single blade of a vane pump.

Hiram Hall, one of the best esophageal speakers the present writer has ever heard, described the tasks as follows:

> It is so simple: The tongue and the fauces pump columns of air down the gullet, just as they do when you want to bring on a belch; only this time you are not intent on belching and you don't. But the belly muscles do contract with more or less sudden sturdiness and the column of air is forced back up and out of the gullet, through its slightly constricted orifice, and the sound (not so gusty) is there. This is your new voice sound which will grow with practice and experience to be as usable as your original voice sound.
>
> And here, a final thought. You know how, in the ordinary act of swallowing, the movements of the several parts blend into a single automatic movement. So, also, you will find in this new act of voice production (by pumping air into and then forcing it out of the gullet) do the movements combine into a single movement. With practice it will become nigh instantaneous. Like the blink of an eye, the parts will go into action and complete the job! The right ones will pump in and the right ones force out air to produce the tones in proper measured pitch, loudness and timbre. And the voice will be there, and the molding of that voice into words and you will say: "God is Good."

It must also be stated here that Hall could also speak by the inhalation method, which he utilized part of the time with little consciousness of so doing.

Tongue pumpers can become very effective speakers. The air is released as it is in the "inhalation" method. Noise is a problem as with all esophageal speech. Not infrequently, each air injection is accompanied by a peculiar low-level sound which is not unlike the words "punk" or "clump." Practice will usually reduce this extraneous noise to a point where it disappears or is barely noticeable.

Learning to speak by method II is facilitated by the use of liquid intake. Soda drinks are desirable if the patient needs a temporary boost after two or three unsuccessful lessons. Pumping air into the top of the esophagus by means of a catheter and rubber syringe bulb can be used in a sort of last-resort effort to give the patient the feel of air below the pseudoglottis. Harrington prefers a warm drink which favors relaxation of the throat, and points out that the mouth and throat can be kept moist by warm drinks, chewing gum, and hard candy. The clinician should recall that the flow of air in and out of the esophagus has a noticeable drying effect on the tissues.

III. The Glossopharyngeal Press or Plosive-injection Method

This promising method had little publicity outside of Holland until the publication in English in 1958 of Damsté's monograph entitled *Oesophageal Speech After Laryngectomy*. During a survey of many speakers in 1956-57 in this country, the author did not find a single speaker of 150 speakers who was aware of using this method. Of course, short of receiving therapy in Holland, anyone using the method would probably be self-taught.

Harrington agrees with this view, stating that method II is the most easily taught, whereas the method under discussion is often adopted, at least in part, by the better speakers without knowledge of how they do it. Harrington and the writer confess their ignorance of the *modus operandi* of this self-taught transition. Probably some completely "spontaneous" or self-taught speakers use method III.

Method III is enthusiastically supported by Damsté and by another eminent speech therapist, Mrs. Mollenaar-Bijl. Damsté (151) has ample radiological and other experimental evidence to support his views.

This system consists of the mouth, tongue, and pharynx which are highly modifiable. In spitting tobacco juice, for example, the press very forcibly pumps liquid. In smoking a pipe, the press pulls away from the air column and creates a relatively strong and well-controlled vacuum. In the laryngectomized patient, the press can also be utilized for blowing the nose, for smelling, and for injecting air into the esophagus.

The writer, although a normal speaker, has no difficulty in injecting air by the "Dutch" method. To get the initial feel of the method, the mouth and tongue are set for the plosive *p,* the cricopharyngeal area is relaxed, and the *p* is directed backward and downward instead of between the lips. Repeating this action will inject considerable air into the esophagus which at first upon release promises only an uncontrolled belch. It should be made clear

that the method just described is primarily for demonstration purposes and to prove that almost no practice is required to get air
into the esophagus.

Damsté (151) recommends the forcible articulation of mono-
syllabic plosive vowel combinations such as *pa, ka,* and *ga.* He recommends further practice with words such as *cartoon* and
pontoon. Both Snidecor and Diedrich are of the opinion that air
intake occurs usually on the first plosive of a word such as "cartoon," and seldom on the second plosive. Damsté's studies indicate
that the esophagus can be replenished before each plosive so that
it never becomes empty.

Diedrich (172), in this country, found that it took fewer air
intakes for plosive sentences (1.5) and more for nonplosive sentences (2.2). He also found that his subjects could phonate about
one and one-half times as long with plosive sentences than with
nonplosive sentences. Diedrich summarizes his view by stating,
"It would appear that plosive sounds are useful in *sustaining*
phonation. In my opinion, they do not completely refill the
esophagus per se." His radiological studies and logic support this
conservative view.

It is noted here that Diedrich and Youngstrom (174) reduce
the methods of air intake to two, that is, "inhalation" and "injection" with "injection" including the act of plosive injection.
Statements of these workers are consonant with the judgment
of the present writer, though terminology is different.

Seeman (666) of Prague, who has dealt with over three hundred laryngectomized patients, maintains that the "Dutch" method is not an injection but rather a "drawing-in" of air into the
expanded esophagus. If such be the case, this drawing in of small
puffs of air is of a very different order than the inhalation method
described as method I. The writer prefers the descriptions of
Damsté, but with the reservation that this injection method is
seldom if ever used exclusively by any one speaker.

However, the writer's confidence in the "Dutch" method is
such that his practice materials are loaded with plosive sounds
with the hope that the speech therapist will do everything possible
to utilize this method for auxiliary air support.

Air Intake—Summary

The present writer, as a speech therapist, prefers to use terminology that allows for the separation of methods into three, and feels obliged to take a stand in regard to these three methods of air intake described above.

1. Initial experimentation with methods I and II appears in order. Methods II and III are rather closely related, and if air pumping proves successful, the injection by plosives follows in logical sequence.

2. The aged and others whose general tonus is low should avoid the inhalation method because it does require substantial expenditure of energy, especially in the learning period.

3. Once a method has been established, the speaker should be encouraged to experiment with other methods, unless in the opinion of the therapist such experimentation would be confusing. One esophageal speaker of the writer's acquaintance was talking with him by the pumping method. He then inhaled two consecutive charges of air and in a louder tone called to a friend in another room, "Hey, Charlie! Get the car!" At least for this speaker, pumping seemed easiest in conversation, whereas a louder tone could be mustered with the inhalation technique.

4. Air, by whatever method, can be taken in very rapidly; one-half of a second seems to be an average value, with some speakers easily cutting this figure in half.

Air Expulsion

There is much more agreement in regard to air expulsion and concomitant voicing than there is in regard to intake of air. For this reason, the writer has chosen to present points of rather general agreement.

1. Physiological breathing and air intake and expulsion are normally synchronized. Inhalation of lung air usually assists the intake of esophageal air, and the exhalation of lung air facilitates the explusion of air from the esophagus. Tracheostomic noise, which accompanies the exhalation of lung air, must be reduced through practice. When we state that breathing and esophageal

charging are synchronous, we depend entirely upon recent radiological and other "breathing" studies rather than upon older opinions which oftentimes stressed a marked separation between the two functions. Damsté (151), and Snidecor and Curry found only generally synchronous behavior, although the latter found an excellent speaker who could, as he said "by a trick," expel esophageal air and speak while inhaling lung air. In this connection, it should be recalled that many normal speakers can speak on inhalation, but again as a trick rather than as a normal performance. Also, it should be noted that Anderson (10) found general synchrony, but lack of it in small detail and in reference to intake of the air in the mouth. As will be noted elsewhere, Isshiki and Snidecor (356), using very sensitive airflow measuring devices, found that air movement is more complex than indicated in previous studies. Suffice it to say here that synchrony is usual with "inhalers," common with tongue pumpers, and not essential to plosive-injectors. This writer contends that all of these methods may be combined in one speaker.

Synchronous movement does not mean that the esophageal speaker necessarily takes or expels a full breath while in the act of charging and releasing air. As a matter of fact, only the general direction of the two movements is the same with, on occasion, several air-charges taken and expelled per full physiological exhalation. In other cases, rather shallow breathing accompanies each air-charge. The writer has known speakers who felt compelled to take a full breath with each air-charge, an act which becomes almost impossible when we recall that even for the superior speaker each air-charge is discharged in only about one and one-half seconds. One such speaker, who was both slow and noisy, breathed so heavily that he seriously hyperventilated and after a minute or two of speech became quite dizzy.

2. The diaphragm is important in air expulsion as well as in air intake, and its action may be rather active especially in loud speech, or more passive in that it can shut off the lower portion of the esophagus retaining the air in the upper portion of the esophagus where it can be utilized.

3. The esophagus itself has an elastic wall. At least before a peristaltic move sets in, the air-filled tube would be like a toy rubber balloon and expel air as a result of its tendency to retain its original condition or constriction.

4. The substantial alveolar pressure in exhalation, in most cases, assisted by the accompanying swelling of the trachea, helps force the air from the esophagus.

5. The air is held briefly in the top half or third of the esophagus of the effective speaker. Most radiological studies support the contention that air is held high in the esophagus, and that there is little of it. With perhaps an average of 9.5 ml per word, even the phrases of the very superior speaker would utilize only about 40 to 70 ml of esophageal air. Proof of greater air use has been uncertain with early instrumentation, although both Kaiser (377) and Voorhoeve (790) demonstrated that air may be in the stomach during speech. With the advantage of recently developed airflow apparatus, Snidecor and Isshiki (711) demonstrated that a superior speaker could expel during speech 615 cc of air over a period of twenty-six seconds. This is three times the volume of the esophagus. It should be noted, however, that this was an "athletic" rather than a usual performance.

6. Voicing is usually in the cricopharyngeal area. A segment as well as the top of the gullet vibrates. Other vibrators are available and sometimes used.

7. All workers seem agreed that relaxation is necessary in order to get air into the top of the esophagus and to release it. It is obvious that there is great variability of tension in release of air, otherwise the expert speaker would be unable to vary his speech by one full octave. Psychophysiological tension, as in anger or fear, usually makes speech impossible.

8. Pushing the head back when releasing air frequently improves loudness and quality, and tends to raise the fundamental pitch.

Chapter XII

Basic Considerations in Learning to Speak Again

JOHN C. SNIDECOR

Who Learns to Speak Again

IT MAY SEEM completely unlikely on first glance that the laryngectomee had any personality differences from the normal prior to his operation. However, Webb and Irving (801), in a lengthy study of seventy-seven male laryngectomees, using in the main Szondian procedures, concluded that (1) most of the laryngectomees manifested the oral triad of excessive speaking, drinking, and smoking; and (2) there were other signs of instability and adjustmental difficulty leading in the direction of asociality (Woltisbuel Index) rather than in the direction of neuroticism. Research in progress by Blake, utilizing methods more precise than Szondian, supports in general the view of Webb and Irving. Webb believes that if there is postoperative shock it is no greater than that which occurs after any other major operation.

Psychological factors are in the main more important than physiological factors when it comes to acquiring a new voice. This recognition is made by Stoll (738) in his description of most of these factors; by Hodson and Oswald (325) through their presentation of successful and unsuccessful cases; and by Fontaine and Mitchell (214) who have given significant attention to problems of anxiety and tension.

Although often exaggerated, the fears held by laryngectomees are based on reasonable assumptions. Stoll lists these as follows:

(1) The fear of the word cancer and the many semantic implications involved in such a word. The fear of death is probably the paramount fear. (2) The fear of operations in general. (3) The fear of the permanent loss of voice. The anxiety associated with this fear results from the assumed consequences of permanent aphonia. The patient's entire pattern of interpersonal relationships built up through the years becomes threatened. He worries about the probable loss of his job, his security, his friends, etc.

The fears often experienced by patients postoperatively are as follows: (1) The fear of the recurrence of the cancer, hence the continued fear of death. (2) Fears due to the new physiological relationships resulting from the laryngectomy. (The inability to lift heavy objects, the breathing and coughing from the tracheal stoma, the often impaired sense of smell and taste, the cosmetic liabilities of the tracheal stoma, etc.). (3) The fear of old age which has been aggravated by the feeling of uselessness resulting from the loss of speech. The depression frequently observed often has its roots in this specific fear. The loss of earning power further contributes to this feeling of uselessness. (4) Fear of being unable to re-establish old patterns of interpersonal relationships. (5) The fears associated with the anticipation of failing to learn a new method of speaking.

Here it should be noted that fear tenses the top of the esophagus just as it does many other body parts and thus inhibits the learning that the laryngectomee fears cannot take place. The process can become cyclical, and it is the clinician's responsibility to break the cycle or see that it never occurs.

The esophageal speaker is frequently one who has a total geriatics problem associated with the specific problem of learning to speak again. Dr. Robert Harrington (309), who has probably taught esophageal speech to as many patients as any other single therapist, expresses his knowledge of the older patient briefly and completely as follows:

> Because he is slower to recuperate, he is slower coming to voice training. This allows a greater period of silence, during which time poor habits of communication may be developed. The older person has weaker muscles, is quicker to fatigue. He is likely to become discouraged because the voice remains weak, and he may use it for only short periods of time. Because of the possibility that either he or his spouse may have reduced hearing acuity, he may be less successful in monitoring his own voice, and less successful in being heard by those in his immediate family. The older person may have masticatory problems associated with denture problems. This may require a soft diet, which in turn will fail to stimulate sufficient pharyngeal and esophageal activity necessary to the development of a satisfactory pseudovoice. Other problems include insufficient economic and social need to talk. Emphasis should be placed on the need for voice training as early as is consistent with general health, stimulating masticatory action, and arranging for social contacts designed to stimulate desire to communicate. In some cases, because of the multiplicity of problems, an instrument would seem to be the method of choice for pseudovoice.

When we study the several authorities who have looked closely at the problem, we must conclude that a certain type of person will most likely learn to speak effectively. First, he will be extroverted, perhaps aggressively so, and socially oriented. Second, his ego will be very much involved in his vocational, professional, and social activities. Stoll points out that the successful speakers expressed themselves well and enjoyed so doing before the operation, and afterward learn to speak intelligibly.

A perusal of case studies abstracted from the Hodson and Oswald (325) English studies, and of the authors in this country, supports the contentions made in the paragraph directly above. From Hodson and Oswald:

1. J. S., male, 31 years. Highly strung, determined man . . . Second treatment said four vowels and one word in oesophageal speech. Capable of fluent speech . . . Spoke for two and one-half minutes before large audience.

2. G. V., male, 52 years. Sheet metal worker. Carcinoma of larynx. A powerfully built man, ex-boxing champion, determined, with keen sense of humour. First day belched well. Said vowels with good oesophageal voice. 5.12.47: No belching. Sentences in loud oesophageal voice. From start was relaxed and used diaphragm well. "Swallows" air before speaking; inclined to gulp when starting to speak. During following year his voice improved steadily but was hampered by air swallowing. 1951: Cineradiography. 26.6.52: Voice excellent. No air swallowing. Easy air intake. Speaks at business firm's committee meetings. Boxes.

3. F. C., male, 42 years. Chaplain. A tough, wiry man; independent and determined. Carcinoma of larynx. Pre-operative treatment: conversed with good oesophageal speakers and had mechanism of voice productions explained to him. 5.5.50: Total laryngectomy (Mr. Myles Fromby). Post-operative fistula developed. 3.7.50: Speech therapy started. Produced belch after a drink. Poor relaxation. 6.7.50: Two words spoken "naturally" without belching. Excellent whisperer. Uses diaphragm well. 17.7.50: Several words spoken in oesophageal voice during a whispered conversation. No belching or air swallowing. 4.9.50: Three or four word phrases in good tone. 23.10.50: Anxiety over future occupation. Patient moved elsewhere; voice deteriorated; and he recommenced "swallowing air." Gradually improved on return to London with regular work and speech treatment. 4.12.50: Enjoying smoking; breathing in and out via nose. Keen sense of smell. 12.1.51: Full time Chaplain — taking services, managing Youth Group; NOT preaching. 9.4.51: Speech very

clean in conversation and over telephone, with good continuity and phrasing. Whistles tunes and sings. 16.7.51: Cineradiography. 21.7.51: Spoke in four languages at a Demonstration — clearly heard. 6.10.52: Preached sermon in Chapel; easily heard at end of Chapel. 25.1.53: Volume and quality of voice improved generally. Preached from pulpit of a Church and heard easily.

Samples from the author's own contacts are reported below:

1. W.M. was 55 years of age when first contacted. He was a clear speaker who benefitted by articulation drill. A teacher of vocal music, he had coached one of the great tenors of the 1920's and 30's and he still led the Choir in a large church. Determined, proud, and a meticulous dresser, he was a cultured extrovert who loved company and conversation.

2. H.H. is a superior speaker, 70 years of age, with ten years of speaking experience. He graduated as a young man from one of the best engineering schools in the nation. He was in turn a successful engineer and an investment banker before his retirement. Even after his laryngectomy this man's manner is such as to dominate in a courteous and natural way most conversational situations.

3. H.C. is a superior speaker, 48 years of age, with a very loud, very clear, but somewhat harsh voice. In one performance he attained 22 syllables, although more usually he performs from the four to eight syllable level. This man has been a house painter all of his life, and one senses that he is, and knows he is, one of the best men in the trade. He learned to speak easily and quickly.

4. R.S. is a satisfactory speaker, 35 years of age, who held an important junior executive position with a large corporation. The father of several children, he both wanted and needed to return to work. He approached esophageal speech in a relaxed yet enthusiastic manner. Six weeks from the initiation of speech therapy he was intelligible.

There is little need to dwell on the failures, but it can be said briefly that the need to speak and the will to speak are usually not present in these cases. The writer remembers a well-to-do business man who, after his laryngectomy, partially retired and then hired a secretary and a valet-chauffeur who could read lips. One patient seen in the hospital only wanted to know if he could keep on drinking.

It is the author's belief that personalities, even at a fairly advanced age, can usually be sufficiently changed to insure attitudes and working habits leading to successful speech. As a matter of fact, a number of men and women have found in Lost Chord Clubs and New Voice Clubs a closer and more meaningful social life than they previously enjoyed.

It is important that the total counseling, guidance, teaching, and social program be considered, for this program can carry many persons to successful speech who otherwise would not have the knowledge, the courage, and the tenacity to achieve it.

1. Most would agree that the patient should be postoperatively counseled by his surgeon and if possible by both a laryngectomee and a speech therapist. The patient should listen to esophageal speech and to an artificial larynx. Some workers would eliminate any contact with esophageal speakers prior to surgery with the thought that this experience is too traumatic. If time allows, the patient should learn to charge air and perhaps vibrate the top of the gullet. He can take in air as easily or more easily with the larynx in place than with it removed. Experimentation with an artificial larynx does no harm and proves that here is a mechanical device which one can fall back on if necessary.

2. As soon as visitors are allowed, they should come. The trauma of the cancer, loss of voice, and fear of death has been severe. The wife, children, the boss, laryngectomees, and the speech therapist should visit.

3. When the patient is released by the surgeon, speech therapy should begin and should be as rigorous as medical judgment allows. This is a critical period during which the family and friends can give a great deal of support, preferably in a straightforward manner.

4. When the patient has mastered sufficient speech to meet simple needs with even low-level efficiency, he should contact, if at all possible, the nearest Lost Chord Club or New Voice Club. He will meet and make friends who have been through the same experience. Most important, he will be encouraged to speak and will be helped in his efforts to speak more effectively. These groups usually invite speech therapists to help them, and they own or otherwise have access to tape recorders and public-address amplifiers.

5. The patient must learn to strive for intelligible speech and

also to accept the fact that his speech will never be perfect. Strangers to esophageal speech will assume that the speaker has a sore throat or a "whiskey voice." However, voice quality should never be sold short. Cooper (130), who has taught many laryngectomees to speak effectively, insists that quality can be emphasized even in very early instruction.

6. The patient should get back on the job or, if he is retired, into his social group as soon as possible.

7. Because the laryngectomy is frequently done in middle or late middle life, the patient and his spouse will have or will soon experience the normal hearing loss associated with advancing years. At the time of the operation, or a few years later, the spouse should wear a hearing aid if he or she is even a marginal candidate for one. The effective esophageal speaker has ample loudness for the normal listener, but he cannot shout. A small amplifier should be used for conferences and comparable speaking situations (Fig. 40), especially when elderly people with hearing losses are to be in the audience. The laryngectomee may wear a denture and not infrequently have a resultant articulation problem.

8. If esophageal speech cannot be learned, then the patient should use an artificial larynx.

Special Problems of Women

In addition to the problems encountered by both sexes are those special problems of women. The problems of 240 women laryngectomees were studied in 1966 by Gardner, and certain differences were obtained between men and women. First, women react with more despondency than do men when threatened with removal of the larynx. Three-fourths of the women were married at the time of surgery and in turn more than three-fourths of these married women were supported by the presence of their husbands when cancer was reported. The picture is not entirely pleasant since two husbands asked for a divorce and one said his business relations would be jeopardized. The total picture, however, favors the married women in regard to support, sympathy, and the ability to face the operation. Directly before the operation, women wished to be counseled by female laryngectomees,

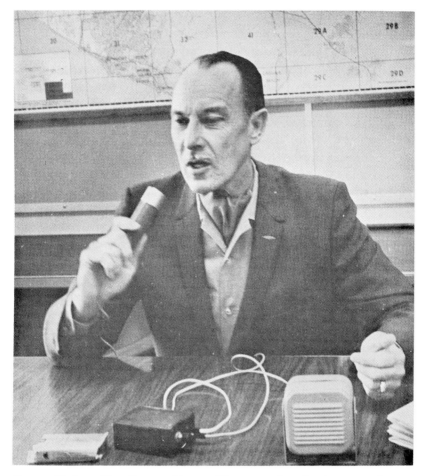

FIGURE 40. A small easily portable amplifier serves in a lecture or conference situation.

and when they were not available, they preferred to write to a female laryngectomee rather than to talk with a male laryngectomee. Counsel from the surgeon is necessary and desirable. Sixty per cent of the women were shocked at their appearances, and several fainted.

Upon returning home, 46 per cent of reporting wives stated their husbands avoided them, pitied them, or babied them too much. Fifty-four per cent wrote about the loyalty of their husbands and their displays of confidence.

Specific to speech, the subjects were somewhat embarrassed at the low pitch of esophageal speech. More married women accepted esophageal speech than did unmarried women. Eighty-two per cent of those with a favorable reaction to speech succeeded, whereas only 64 per cent of those with unfavorable reactions succeeded. Two-thirds of the wives were assisted in speech by husbands, by such acts as taking them to speech classes and bringing visitors to the home. It proved a common complaint that esophageal speech was not easily understood. This, in some cases, was due to the fact that spouses were at an age where hearing had been lost.

Women insisted that laryngectomees should be taught by trained teachers. Determination was essential in learning, and affection and confidence were important. The importance of motivation and self-discipline was stressed. One woman worked hard to give her sons and grandchildren her new voice as a Christmas present. One woman very wisely identified herself over the telephone so that she would not be called "Sir." Effective speakers emphasized that working women should return to employment as soon as possible and speech would improve thereby. More than half of the women returned to work after surgery. Successful job holders advised others to " (1) Dress neatly; (2) cover the stoma with an attractive scarf, bib or lacy material; (3) return to work as soon as possible; (4) keep in mind that with good speech there should be no employment problem."

All in all, the person learns to speak who most wants and needs to speak. We are not all outgoing and socially oriented, but most of us can learn to speak again for our own satisfaction and that of others.

It can be seen from the above discussion that we must consider the laryngectomee as a *whole* person excepting only his lack of vocal cords. K. J. Knepflar (398) calls this approach "individualized speech therapy." His evaluation form, which takes into account this concept, is printed below. The numbers in parentheses indicate the number of blank lines normally needed in developing a case study.

Speech Therapy Evaluation Form For Laryngectomized Patients

Name   Age   Date
Address   Phone
Source of Referral

1. Operative Factors
    Date (s) of surgery (1)
    Extent of surgery (3)
    Postoperative complications (2)
    Irradiation (2)
2. Physical Factors
    General physical condition (2)
    Spread of cancer (2)
    Upper respiratory conditions (2)
    Other physical factors (3)
3. Geriatric Factors (4)
4. Auditory Factors
    Audiometric results (3)
    Comments (3)
5. Emotional Factors
    Depression (1)
    Motivation (2)
    Degree of dependency (1)
    Acceptance of esophageal speech (2)
    Other personality traits or problems (2)
6. Social Factors
    Educational background (1)
    Cultural background (1)
    Patient's sociability (2)
    Family attitudes (3)
    Vocational aspects (1)
7. Intellectual Factors (3)
8. Articulation Factors
    Motor factors (1)
    Dental factors (1)
    Accuracy of articulation (2)
    Foreign accent (2)
9. Language Factors
    Language comprehension (3)
    Language usage (3)
Summary of pertinent factors (3)
Apparent prognosis (2)
Recommendations (4)

Who Is Your Teacher?

There has been considerable discussion in regard to this question and some disagreement in regard to the answers. However, the opinion of the present writer is that the individual should be initially instructed by a speech pathologist. *Members of the*

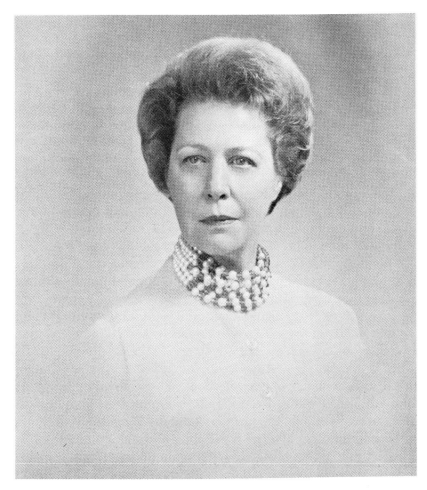

FIGURE 41. Several strands of beads serve as an artistic shield for the stoma. (*Courtesy of Brooks Photography, Bethesda, Md.*)

American Speech and Hearing Association Available for Referral of Laryngectomees is the title of a publication issued by the American Cancer Society in 1964. It may be obtained either from the IAL or the American Speech and Hearing Association. (See Appendix, "Directory of Sources of Supply.") Speech pathologists will normally enter into the teaching situation without prejudice concerning the way in which the individual should inject and use air. It is also to be noted that the speech pathologist will, in all probability, have psychological training so that he may counsel with both the laryngectomized individual and family members. He also may be in a very favorable position of going "to bat" for the laryngectomee with his employer. The nature of the operation can be explained to the employer, and it can be noted that speech, if once established, will gradually become more fluent and intelligible. Emphasis can be given to the fact that the individual remains physically and intellectually capable, and that he may be even more motivated than he had been in the past.

However, the assistance of laryngectomees is essential to effective instruction. A surgeon with whom this writer works desires that a laryngectomized individual who is a good speaker visit an individual prior to his operation. On occasion, he has asked that I do the same thing. Once speech is even partially established, the laryngectomized adjunct is essential to the training program. However, I wish to initiate phonation and develop a pattern of speech prior to the client's close and continuous contact with another esophageal speaker. With good luck, this may only take a week or two. When at least a temporary speech pattern is established, I want the new esophageal speaker to contact individuals that I know will be compatible with him or her. A New Voice Club or Lost Chord Club may be just what the individual needs if such a club is available. However, it must be remembered that many work outside the metropolitan areas and have available only a few esophageal speakers who have not found it practical to organize themselves into a club.

Rehabilitation Resources

At all times the speech therapist and the patient should be aware of rehabilitation resources in the community. In general these will include:

1. A local or regional branch of the American Cancer Society.
2. A local, regional, or state university or college with a speech and hearing center.
3. A branch of the International Association of Laryngectomees (IAL) See Appendix "Sources of Supply."

4. The American Speech and Hearing Association, 90030 Old Georgetown Road, Washington, D. C. 20014.
5. The state office for vocational rehabilitation. (The title of this office will vary from state to state, and offices will not be available in small cities. These offices are to be contacted when the patient's vocation must be changed.)

Chapter XIII

Speech Therapy for Those with Total Laryngectomy

John C. Snidecor

PRECEDING CHAPTERS have established the research and clinical background for practice in voice which can begin as soon as the physician releases the patient for speech therapy. At the time the speech therapist first sees the patient, he will very likely be in poor physical condition for speech rehabilitation. With good surgery and good luck, the fifth recurrent laryngeal nerve still supplies innervation to the top portion of the esophagus, but the patient will not have learned to utilize this potentially useful signal. Through speech, air, soda water, sour drinks, hot coffee, coarse food, and so forth, he can become more conscious of his new glottis.

The entire muscular mechanism, upon which new speech by any esophageal method depends, will usually be weak and flaccid by reason of the use of soft and liquid foods before, during, and even after the hospital stay. If dentures are worn, the problem may be compounded. The patient must learn as quickly as possible to chew and swallow a "normal" diet of unground meat, cooked and uncooked vegetables, nonmushy cereals, and the like. A not-too-tender steak cut into moderately small pieces, raw carrots, raw celery, raisins, peanuts, and Grape-Nuts℗ are examples of desirable foods. Obviously the patient will stay within any dietary limitations set by his physician. Harrington (309) is so firmly convinced of the need for muscular tonus that he will not accept a patient until he is actually on a full and normal diet. In searching for experimental subjects and in normal social relationships, the author has dined with dozens of esophageal speakers, and every effective speaker ate a normal meal — usually with gusto.

It is well at this point for the therapist to remind himself again of the psychological problems faced by the patient. These are covered comprehensively in Chapter XII under Who Learns to Speak Again?. Specifically and personally, some of these problems were communicated to the writer by the late Laurance W. Phelps, who was not of retirement age when he became a laryngectomee. Told in the third person to the writer, it is a story of a man who was helped by his surgeon, his speech therapist, his employer, and most of all by himself.

He is a structural engineer who has nine years service with an engineering construction firm previous to his laryngectomy.

When he returned to his former position, he knew that it was imperative that he should learn to speak again as soon as possible. He couldn't envision holding his position without being able to speak. His duties with the company require that he deal with draftsmen, estimators, field superintendents, salesmen, material men, etc. Also, he gives expert testimony in court cases.

He contacted a speech therapist immediately after his return to work and started speech lessons daily. At the time he was learning to talk, it was thought that daily lessons were beneficial — now lessons are spaced apart so as to give the student adequate time for practice between lessons.

After a few lessons, he thought it was necessary to learn faster. He borrowed a speaking device which he demonstrated to his employer. The employer was not pleased with the device. He said that the progress of esophageal speech was satisfactory and that there was no necessity for the device. Furthermore, he said that he would rather have the employee in the office without being able to say a single esophageal word than to see him use the device. He said that soon the employee would speak well. This encouragement and praise was greatly appreciated by the employee. The employer was so considerate that the employee was obliged to regain his speech quickly. Moreover, he accepted the challenge of learning to speak with much enthusiasm. Therefore, the employee went to work with renewed energy in order to speed up the progress for the benefit of the company as well as for himself.

The employee followed the speech therapist's instructions implicitly by practicing long hours and by observing the required rest periods between the practice periods. One day after speech had returned to the laryngectomee, the employer told the employee that he or no one else in the company considered the new speech a handicap. The employee has fulfilled his position with the same employer for eleven years since the laryngectomy. Some time ago he joined the International Toastmasters Club and takes his turn speaking the same as the rest of the members.

It is not the intention of the writer to discredit the use of speaking devices — he realizes that in some cases they are essential. However, he feels that the laryngectomee should give esophageal speech a fair trial and should consult his speech therapist and his surgeon before resorting to a speaking device. Esophageal speech is considered to be better than the use of mechanical devices because it is more practical and can't be misplaced or lost. It must be a terrible feeling to need a device in a hurry and not be able to find it.

Laryngectomees are proud of their new voices and are grateful for the encouragement that they receive from interested parties. They are happy with their accomplishment which has come after many, many hours of prolonged but necessary practice. It should be kept in mind that study under the supervision of a speech therapist is essential in order to develop good esophageal speech.

We suggest that the patient read the above-stated case of Phelps, and the cases of Hall and Green in Chapter I.

With encouragement from these three cases, and if possible, from some new larynegtomee friends, the patient is ready to go to work. However, the therapist is not ready to go to work until he reminds himself of the responsibility which he has for working toward the development of a usable, intelligible, and pleasing voice. Morton Cooper (130) summarizes these goals as follows:

> The voice of the laryngectomized patient is sadly in need of the vocal rehabilitation efforts we afford the functional and organic voice disorders, such as nodes, polyps, contact ulcer, and myasthenia laryngis. Too often, the patient's demand for speech is abetted by those therapists who have little time, little patience, and little concern for a pleasing, well-modulated quality in the esophageal voice. The aphonic or severe dysphonic whom we see is in no way thought to have terminated therapy because a moderate dysphonia now exists. Rather, we continue our vocal rehabilitation efforts until the voice is clear, easy, and well-modulated. But, for the laryngectomized patient, we have no such goals at the outset of therapy. Often we neglect to afford a quality voice, or development of quality in voice for the laryngectomized. It is my view that quality is the essence and not a refinement that should be afforded the laryngectomized patient. Quality should be established at the beginning and not at the conclusion of therapy, since few patients are willing to develop a good voice once they have acquired some form of esophageal voice. We should not rush the patient into voice, but into an understanding of how to produce an efficient and well-modulated voice at the outset of therapy. It may slow down therapy at the beginning, and frustrate the patient not to

speak earlier or faster, but the final result is much better and a goal to be sought, if excellence is sought.

In the first formal contact with the new laryngectomee, three appointments are set up for the first day. These are scheduled for early morning, mid-morning, and mid-afternoon. The establishment of three appointments for the first day is of importance because a number of our clients must travel a considerable distance. Even more important than the convenience factor is the advantage that may come from phonation during the first day of instruction. Usually phonation is achieved during one of three meetings. When this occurs, the client is sent home with practice exercises. The importance of gaining phonation on the first day of teaching can be overemphasized, but if phonation is possible the client's morale is improved, and this state of mind is transferred to the family especially if the laryngectomee can go home and use even a simple word or two. Daily or tri-weekly appointments are deemed essential until basic speech habits are established.

The main objective during the first stage of learning is to voice vowel and vowel-plus-plosive consonants. The writer places great stress on combining these two classes of sounds because Damsté's studies and, more recently, Diedrich's (172) x-rays seem to prove beyond any doubt that plosive consonants can, at the very least, help considerably in charging the esophagus with air.

At this point the writer recommends that each patient be supplied with the manual and training recordings produced by Melvin Hyman or Mary Doehler (see Appendix, Sources of Supply). These are not do-it-yourself kits, but important listening aids for those attempting to establish a new voice.

The Nine Stages of Development

The therapist may now consider the stages as stated below as representing levels of achievement rather than lessons as such. Patients do not fit exact patterns, so we choose not to prescribe in great detail.

1. Get air in — get air out. This is obviously the most basic act of new speech. Experiment with air-intake methods as described in Chapter XI on charging and expulsion of air. The air intake should be immediately followed by the speech sound. Harrington, in discussing the tongue-pumping or swallowing method, states, "I encourage a hard, fast swallow so that the gulp will be a definite land mark — after which he quickly produces sound. Gulp is later reduced by slowing speed of air intake." Always with women and often with men the present writer uses the concept of *sniff-inject-pah* proposed by Diedrich. This method combines in one continuous movement tongue pumping and plosive injection. Even when some liquid is required, it is placed on the tip of the tongue and the word "inject" is used. As we have previously noted, the action is not that of a swallow, and so that term should not be used. With the strong extroverted male, this writer frequently used the forced-belch method. It depends on the old habit of sucking air in to release gas or air in the stomach. (See previous detailed descriptions.) No matter what method is used, *in quick — out quick* is essential for effective speech. Reference to Chapter V on time and rate will uncover ample evidence for our insistence on this technique. Produce any vowel. *Ah* is as good as any, but *ē* and *ō* are almost as easy (pah, pay, poh) .

2. *Produce consonants (plosives), and vowels, and diphthongs.* At this stage, use lots of plosive sounds but do not be concerned about how carefully they are made. (Samples: tea, tah, bee, cow, pet, cat, bag, boy, bow, bib, pay, toy, Bob.)

3. *Voice simple, useful, one-syllable words.* (Samples: hi, yes, no, find, good, boy, girl, tree, red, bread. One, two, three, four, five, six, se/ven, eight, nine, ten.)

4. *Voice two-syllable words — at first with one air-charge per syllable, then with one air-charge for both syllables.* (Samples: summer, winter, hotter, colder, coffee, butter, breathing, calling, breakfast, luncheon, dinner.)

5. *Voice simple phrases with one charge if possible.* (Samples: It's dinner time. Don't forget him. Buy some gum. He came on time. It cost too much. Mail the cards.)

When speech becomes marginally useful, the patient's image of his own speech is clarified by the use of a recording device. Cooper (136) describes its use.

One method of improving the concept of what the patient is producing is the playback of the patient's sound as compared to the therapist's sound. Listening to the tape playback, the patient can compare his tone with that produced by the therapist; then the diffusiveness that exists may be eliminated by ear training and vocal practice.

Patients have commented: "I don't realize how it sounds without the tape machine" or "It is very helpful to hear how I sound compared to you." Playback of the patient's tone is useful and very necessary to acquire a good sense of tone and a good tone.

At this point, it must be emphasized that effective phrasing should be learned before loudness is attempted. Gradually try to work up to a minimum of three to five words or more if possible without consideration for loudness. Sufficient loudness can be achieved later, and it will frequently result naturally and easily from good phrasing and clear speech which is discussed directly below.

6. Practice articulation and connected speech with emphasis on (a) vowels, (b) diphthongs, and (c) consonants. Given reasonable loudness and quality, intelligibility or understandability is almost entirely a result of effective articulation. Articulation refers to the movement of the speaking mechanism. It follows that the articulators are those parts of the speech mechanism that move or are moved against. The tongue is a moving articulator, whereas the teeth and the roof of the mouth are static articulators. Effective work from the moving articulators is essential for clear speech.

The case for clear articulation is especially important to the esophageal speaker for two rather obvious reasons. First, the basic phonation of the cricopharyngeus can never be as clear as the voice from a normal larynx, so the vowels, semi-vowels, and diphthongs must be articulated with a reasonable amount of extra care. Second, the consonants, with especial reference to the unvoiced (whispered) consonants, are formed in large part from buccal (mouth) and pharyngeal (throat) air, and the amount of air available is of course substantially less than that from a normal air stream.

It is fortunate that improvement in articulation is not difficult once basic voice has been mastered. Some esophageal speakers intuitively realize the importance of clear tongue, mouth, and lip movements and speak so clearly and naturally that their lips are easy for the deaf to read.

A systematic approach to articulation speeds one's efforts toward clear, effective speech and at the same time continues air-charge practice which is of the greatest importance.

a. Vowel Practice. There are an even dozen vowels in common use in General American Speech. If you live in the Deep South or down East, you may add or subtract a vowel or two but, in all parts of the country, mastery of these twelve vowels will suffice.

In addition to a reasonably good vocal vibration, there are two factors that make for clear vowel production. First, the high point of the tongue should be in the proper position for the vowel in question. Second, the lips should be properly shaped. The diagram, with its brief explanation, demonstrates both of these factors.

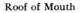

Roof of Mouth

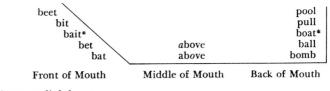

beet		pool
bit		pull
bait*		boat*
bet	*above*	ball
bat	above	bomb

| Front of Mouth | Middle of Mouth | Back of Mouth |

*At times are diphthongs.

The front vowels from *ē* downward require a gradual lowering of the tongue and dropping of the jaw. Most important is lip position, which is slit-like in *ē,* gradually progressing to a rather large oval in the vowel in *bat.*

The two middle vowels have a neutral sound, and the tongue is in a neutral, relaxed position. The mouth opening is small.

The back vowels from *ū* downward require a gradual lowering of the tongue and jaw. Most important is the rounded lip shape for the top back vowels which becomes less rounded as one progresses toward the lower vowels.

Practice the following pairs of words using, wherever possible, one air-charge for each pair. Try to make each vowel stand out as a perfect example of its kind. For the time being, pay little attention to the consonants.

bit	beat	pull	pool	deed	did
bait	bit	poke	pull	did	date
bet	bait	ball	boat	debt	pat
bat	bet	bob	ball	pat	putt
but	bat			tool	took
				book	coke
				poke	tall
				pawed	pod
				cod	cud

b. Diphthong Practice. There are five diphthongs in General American Speech. Again, if you live down South or down East, certain acceptable differences in your speech will exist.

The five common diphthongs are those in the words *low, cow, pail, pie,* and *toy.* The sounds *ā* and *ō,* with slight variations, may be vowels or diphthongs. Diphthongs are two vowels in a smooth blend with the stress on the first vowel. The tongue moves upward for the second vowel, and the mouth opening is smaller for the second vowel.

It can be said with confidence that anyone who can make the separate vowels in a diphthong can make the diphthong. Nevertheless, these vowel combinations contribute to intelligibility and they should be practiced as carefully as the vowels.

Practice the following pairs of words using, whenever possible, one air-charge for each pair. Make each diphthong stand out as a perfect example of its kind. Stress the first vowel and relax the second.

toe	cow	plow	go
bough	bay	day	gown
pay	pie	buy	jay
guy	boy	toy	kite

c. Consonant Practice. There are twenty-three consonants in General American Speech. With the addition of the combination sounds *ch* and *j,* there are, for all practical purposes, twenty-five consonants to be practiced. The *h* sound causes a great deal of discussion among esophageal speakers. Some contend it can be made, and others state flatly that this particular sound cannot be

made. As a plain matter of fact, *h* is the only true glottal or laryngeal consonant in the English language and cannot be made in
anything approximating a normal manner after the larynx has
been removed. Some speakers create a point of friction in the back
of the throat and form a substitute sound for *h*. This particular
sound contributes very little to intelligibility, and it is the writer's
feeling that any concern with *h* should be postponed until all of
the other consonants have been mastered. Eleven of these are considerably more difficult than the remaining fourteen, and the
exercises given below stress work on these intrinsically difficult
sounds.

Reasonable loudness and clarity of voice and vowels are not
enough for good intelligibility. Research by Bell Telephone,
World War II Studies, and a great deal of individual research
indicate the need for effective consonant articulation and for the
concomitant need for good instruments to carry consonants by
wire or air.

John O. Anderson (10) found the voiceless consonants difficult in esophageal speech, and so they merit careful practice — but
always with a vowel or diphthong before or after the consonant.
Combining the findings of Anderson and Hyman, and general-
izing slightly, we find that vowels are the easiest of speech sounds
and that final consonants are more difficult than initial consonants. From easy to difficult are the affricates, laterals, glides,
nasals, plosives, and fricatives. Parenthetically, we should note
that diphthongs are a combination of vowels and obviously are in
the easy group of speech sounds for esophageal speakers.

All of the exercises given in this section are developed in keep-
ing with the Anderson and Hyman studies as well as being based
on certain well-established information on general intelligibility.

The esophageal speaker forms the consonants in large part
with buccal (mouth) and pharyngeal (throat) air. The voiced
consonants are formed in the same manner as the voiceless consonants, except that these sounds are also supported by voicing
from the esophagus.

You will have noted that from the first we have insisted upon
the use of consonants with vowels in voice practice, but the point

has been made that no great attention should be given to these consonants when one first begins to speak again.

Serious practice on the consonants should begin with the unvoiced consonants, and then only after voice has been well-established. Any reversal of this order might encourage the fixation of the whisper habit which is difficult to break.

In forming consonants, air is trapped in the mouth and pharynx and released in a normal fashion for each of the consonants. Because less air is available than was the case with lung air, minor exaggerations in sound formation are in order. For example, with the normal speaker the friction consonant *sh* consumes a good deal of breath. The esophageal speaker does not have the breath to waste, so he can draw the teeth closer together and produce an acceptable sound with less air. Experimentation with difficult sounds will be needed.

Practice on consonants must be approached in perspective. Good clear voicing and satisfactory vowel production are the essence of esophageal speech. Effective consonant articulation is like frosting on the cake — important, but not to be applied until the cake is baked.

Practice the following voiceless plosive consonants in combination with the open vowel. Relax the top of the esophagus and attempt to let each plosive charge the gullet with a small amount of air. It is not critical if you fail to charge air in this, the "Dutch," manner, but it should be remembered that this auxiliary method of charging air is easy on you and your listeners.

pa	pa	pa	ap	ap	ap	apa	apa	apa
ta	ta	ta	at	at	at	ata	ata	ata
ka	ka	ka	ak	ak	ak	aka	aka	aka

Practice the following voiceless fricative or friction sounds. Usually you will need to restrict the air passage more than you did when you had normal breath.

fa	fa	fa	af	af	af	afa	afa	afa
tha	tha	tha	ath		ath	atha	atha	atha
sa	sa	sa	as	as	as	asa	asa	asa
sha	sha	sha	ash	ash	ash	asha	asha	asha
ha	ha	ha	(Not found in			aha	aha	aha

(Not found in
the final
position. Read
text for lack
of importance
of this sound.)

Practice the *wh* glide as if it were a fricative sound.

| wha | wha | wha | (Not found in the final position.) | awha | awha | awha |

Practice the following voiced plosive sounds remembering that these and their accompanying vowel sounds require voicing. The top of the esophagus vibrates.

ba	ba	ba	ab	ab	ab	aba	aba	aba
da	da	da	ad	ad	ad	ada	ada	ada
ga	ga	ga	ag	ag	ag	aga	aga	aga

Practice the following voiced fricative or friction sounds.

va	va	va	av	av	av	ava	ava	ava
tha	tha	tha	ath	ath	ath	atha	atha	atha
za	za	za	az	az	az	aza	aza	aza
zha*	zha	zha	azh	azh	azh	azha	azha	azha

Practice *w* as if it were a fricative.

| wa | wa | wa | (Not found in the final position.) | awa | awa | awa |

Practice the following sounds just to complete the list. No serious problems should be involved.

ma	ma	ma	am	am	am	ama	ama	ama
na	na	na	an	an	an	ana	ana	ana
ang	ang	ang						
ya	ya	ya	(Not found in the final position.)	aya	aya	aya

*zh is pronounced as the *s* in the word *treasure*.

For a final development of clear consonant articulation, practice the following sentences which give emphasis to those American-English consonants that are generally considered relatively difficult to produce, and which also contribute greatly to intelligibility. Also included are the few special sounds which are easy for normal speakers but which are difficult for esophageal speakers.

1) Your speech will be more nearly perfect if you remember that to be hurried is never right.
2) Most people will say "Hello" if you only smile and wave.
3) It was once thought that both a larynx and breath were necessary for speech, but now we know other paths and air sources are usable.
4) The laryngectomee can speak successfully, but to sing most songs is impossible.

5) To speak with ease one must pause often between phrases.
6) One should shape his mouth surely and exactly to make sharp consonants.
7) Few speakers find it easy at first to say "fifty-five."
8) Never give your voice a chance to fatigue.
9) It is usual to think of speech as a pleasurable part of most occasions.
10) If you cannot say "which" and "when," it is permissable to say "witch" and "wen."
11) We make the suggestion that you check your pitch level with your teacher.
12) There is no magic jump to good speech at any age.

7. Stress is achieved by changes in loudness, pitch, quality, and time. For our purposes, we will consider only the important factors of loudness and pitch, for with shifts in loudness and pitch one's voice will never sound monotonous.

We have always assumed that the esophageal speaker could vary the loudness of his voice, but only recently Snidecor and Curry (709) discovered that his pitch could be almost as variable as that of the normal speaker.

At first, some beginning speakers can get the idea of pitch change by a slight postural shift such as raising the chin or pulling the head back a little. Such changes appear to increase the tension at the top of the epiglottis and thus raise pitch. Relaxation will lower pitch.

The sentences given below will serve as sample drills for stress. Make the word in capital letters loud and higher in pitch. See Hyman (345) (*How to Speak Again*) and Fairbanks (200) for additional drills on stress.

    a. I said NO.
    b. He ATE like a pig.
    c. I say you are CRAZY.
    d. Little pitchers have BIG EARS.
    e. NO ONE is going to cheat ME.
    f. He would rather PLAY than work.
    g. DON'T get mad.
    h. It's UNDER the table.
    i. KICK him out.
    j. She LOVES big hats.

8. Use active conversation. This stage is achieved satisfactorily only after the seven previous stages have been reached. Sample questions will bring out answers which cannot be read and prepared for. Active conversation is often a big jump from reading even rather complicated sentences.

Answer the following sample questions.

  a. How are you today?
  b. What is your address?
  c. Are you working now?
  d. What is your most-liked food?
  e. Where would you most like to live?

9. The achievement of satisfactory rate usually results along with the mastery of the previous eight stages.

Check your rate. If you are too slow, practice by reading simple, continuous passages of prose or poetry.

Read the passage stated below as if to a small audience, timing yourself in seconds. Directly below the passage, you will find a table from which you can read your rate in words per minute. The ratings from adequate to very superior are for experienced speakers.

Your rate of speech will be satisfactory if it is as slow as eighty-five words per minute or as rapid as one hundred and forty words per minute. One hundred and twenty words per minute is excellent for superior esophageal speech. It is necessary to take many more pauses for "breath" than does the normal speaker, but these pauses are often less than one-half second in length. You "breathe" for speech more quickly than he does, and use each air-change for from two to five words or even more. He uses his breath for an average of twelve or thirteen words, and his normal rate of speech is about one hundred and sixty-six words per minute.

Seconds	Words per Minute	
120	60	
110	65	—adequate
100	72	
90	80	—good
80	90	
70	103	—excellent
60	120	
50	144	—very superior

To compensate for some of the weaknesses inherent in esophageal speech, procedures may be followed which will be of considerable day-to-day assistance: (a) When it is necessary to converse under conditions of noise, stand close to your listener. (b) When using the telephone, hold the microphone close (lower lip brushing the phone). (c) Women should identify themselves when calling, for example, "This is Mary Jones. . . ." This cancels out the possibility of being called "Sir." (d) If the spouse is hard-of-hearing, he or she should investigate the possibilities of a hearing aid.

Most esophageal speakers will be satisfied, or more than satisfied, if they have mastered the materials of instruction that we have covered up to this point. A few additional suggestions may be in order. Improvement in quality will come, as we have already noted, through continuous and concentrated attention to the proper voicing of vowels and diphthongs. Changing the neck position often influences pitch and loudness. Believe it or not, many esophageal speakers can learn to sing a song. If you really wish to "frost the cake," you may care to practice some of the exercises stated below for increasing frequency or pitch variability.

a. Practice singing a familiar song such as "Pop Goes the Weasel" or "Mary Had a Little Lamb." Other simple melodies will come to mind.
b. Start with your "base" or average note which will probably be about the second C below middle C, and then work up and down the piano scale. Change neck and jaw position to see if these postural changes help.
c. Higher pitch and greater intensity are related in both the normal and the esophageal speaker. If you try for greater loudness, you will almost surely raise your pitch. Conversely, if you try for a higher pitch, you will tend to increase your loudness or intensity.

Shipp (684) has pointed out that these higher pitches are preferred by listening panels.

Chapter XIV

Speech Therapy for Subtotal Laryngectomy and Related Cases

John C. Snidecor

THE SPEECH THERAPIST is seeing an increasing number of cases with subtotal laryngectomy by reason of earlier diagnosis and greatly improved surgical techniques. Most of these cases are men because of the greater incidence of cancer of the larynx among men. Women will occasionally be referred or seek help on their own because of thyroidectomies which at times result in a partial paralysis of the larynx.

When released and referred by the surgeon, this writer desires a report from the surgeon and if possible an examination with the surgeon so that he can point out the nature and extent of the operation and make suggestions for therapy. By way of example, two of us examined the larynx of a young woman who had spent five years and almost twice as many thousands of dollars preparing for a career in teaching. A paralyzed vocal cord and resulting dysphonia suddenly threatened her career and resulted in a severe depression. Fortunately, for purposes of voice therapy, the paralyzed cord was quite spastic. A rationale for therapy was developed, and within nine months the patient was teaching. She has no difficulty in a normal classroom situation but does resort to a portable loud speaker for lecture situations involving audiences of fifty or more, or when talking to smaller groups under noisy conditions.

When the nonoperating vocal cord is not in firm opposition to the "live" cord, laryngologists increasingly use either silicone or Teflon® injections to firm up the paralyzed cord so that it may be contacted by the usable cord. Silicone is most often used either as a trial run before Teflon is injected or may be used in those cases in which one anticipates return of cord function. Teflon, because of its greater stability in the tissue, is used when permanent "pillowing" of the cord is desired and when it is improbable that vocal-cord function will return. Dramatic success is often obtained by these new surgical techniques. Speech therapy, when needed, will follow established methods, some of which are mentioned below.

Cases of the general type under discussion are usually much easier to deal with than are those with total laryngectomy. The air stream is usually relatively unaffected, and so one concentrates on developing new phonatory methods with a speech mechanism that, although often markedly modified, is nevertheless far less drastically altered than it is with those who have experienced a total laryngectomy.

No highly generalized prescription can be written for these patients, but certain fundamental considerations must be taken into account in an appropriate analytical manner. Subsequent to analysis, voice therapy is developed and should in most cases extend over a period of several months.

The Vibrator

The first question to ask is, "What vibrator will be used?" Generally speaking, this is decided with the surgeon, but subsequent experimentation may be necessary. The vocal lips, or what remains of them are the preferred vibrators, and initial dysphonia or even aphonia should not be considered as discouraging unless known limiting factors preclude the use of the vocal lips. A great deal of vocal exercise and trial-and-error approaches are essential before one gives up the use of "normal" vibrators. Above the larynx one has use of the false vocal cords and other potential vibrators. The writer observed with C. Hanley (303), a twelve-year-old boy who had been born without a vestige of vocal cords yet who spoke intelligibly in a low-pitched, hoarse, and rather loud voice. The false vocal cords were the apparent vibrators. A number of years ago the writer observed a seven-year-old boy who had a clear normal voice pitched at approximately 256 Hz, which is the usual level for either girls or boys of this age. In addition, the boy had a relatively clear voice pitched at approximately 136 Hz, or at the level of a mature male voice. Examination of the vocal cords indicated that they were much too short for the lower vibration. No certain determination of the 136-Hz vibrator was made, but probably the false vocal folds were in action. It is of incidental interest to note that this boy used his low voice to "scare his sister" and on Halloween to "scare all the children."

Scores of other cases can be found and described. Suffice it to say that in most cases breath-driven vibrators can be found. If not, esophageal speech or the artificial larynx may be utilized.

Relaxation and Tonal Attack

There is a general agreement that overall physical relaxation is needed in voice cases. There is no doubt but that general physical and psychological tensions are transmitted to the vocal cords. One expression of tension may be excessive and hard closure of the vocal folds which precedes vocalized sound. Even with one vocal cord inoperative, or perhaps even as a result of this condition, many speakers falsely sense that tension will initiate satisfactory phonation. What the speaker gets is a strained, harsh, often high-pitched tone which not only sounds tense but which may be observed as tense by watching the front of the neck for expressions of overt tension. To initiate phonation, the prolonged syllables *gah. . .* and *kah. . .* made in a relaxed fashion will often start easy, relatively nonbreathy phonation in cases where only one cord is operating.

Pitch Level

In no single class of cases is optimal pitch level more important than it is with most of these patients. The new vibratory system, usually with limited efficiency, demands careful pitch placement; at times, shifts upward or downward during therapy are in order until the most efficient level has been found and established. However, pitch variety, as distinguished from pitch level, should not be overemphasized unless it can clearly be shown that variety is possible with the new vibrators.

Achieving a satisfactory pitch level is the result of experimentation. There is no evidence that methods established for the normal voice give much assistance. The writer has used a modification of the method developed by Fairbanks (200), Pronovost, and Snidecor. The subjects will usually have no falsetto, or at times appear to be all falsetto, and will usually have a very narrow pitch range. One-third of the way up to the total pitch range serves as a basis for trial and proves better than no method of approximation. "Singing" up and down with the piano may assist in determining a new pitch level. All trials should be made when the subject is rested and relatively relaxed.

Procedures of fixing pitch level are well known to the experienced therapist and need no discussion here.

Articulation

There are two major contributors to intelligibility, loudness and articulation (movements of the speaking mechanism). When loudness is limited by physiological problems, then articulation which is precise and correctly timed will contribute to intelligibility and even to voice quality itself. We would include both vowel and consonant articulation.

Rate of Speech

It should be obvious that one cannot attend relaxation, new pitch levels, and clear articulation while speaking at a high rate of speech. Darley's (159) mean for normal speakers of 160 words per minute is much too fast for the cases under consideration. On the other hand most, if not all, can speak at 144 to 155 words per minute which would put them at an acceptable rate according to Franke's norms.

Establishing Vocal Efficiency: Duration, Quality, and Loudness

If at all possible, optimum pitch level should be established before extensive drill begins on vocal efficiency. The voices of which we speak are often notably inefficient with huskiness, hoarseness, harshness, and breathiness commonly heard. Breathiness is by far the most common and usually the best indicator of inefficiency. The individual with the inefficient voice must be motivated, directed, and in a sense "forced" in the direction of the efficient voice. In severe cases, such a program frequently takes weeks or months.

Several basic exercises related to all aspects of vocal inefficiency may be of help. It is highly important that a record of each exercise be kept and studied, and usually the record should be shared with the patient.

1. Phonate each one of the vowels and record the time in seconds.
2. Read aloud for checking purposes, always at the same rate and loudness, simple propositional prose such as the "Rainbow Passage" (200). Time each reading in seconds. Keep a record of the number of breaths needed for the passage.
3. Using reading materials in which a line-by-line word count has been established, read as many words as possible per breath and record the results. A moderately slow rate of speaking will be found best. The legato manner should be emphasized.
4. Count as high as possible on each of three breaths. Average the results and record.

The experienced therapist will note that the above exercises should implicity take into account duration, quality, loudness, and rate; he will also have no difficulty devising additional exercises suited to individual needs.

If poor breathing habits are a problem above and beyond vibrator inefficiency they must be dealt with as additional and related problems.

As we have previously noted, if intelligibility is not achieved through exercises in phonation, articulation drill may be in order. All of the purely vocal exercises in Chapter XIII for the esophageal speaker may be utilized, especially with the very inefficient voice.

It is too much to expect that a new voice will emerge and be utilized throughout the day. It should be concentrated upon during all practice periods, with or without the therapist. Gradually, the new voice can be used in more easy, relaxed situations as, for example, in talking to a friend on the telephone, or when reading a story aloud to children or grandchildren. Eventually, total use may be possible.

Chapter XV

The Artificial Larynx

JOHN C. SNIDECOR

IN THE TWENTIETH CENTURY and until a few years ago, surgeons and speech therapists were somewhat overenthusiastic concerning the relative numbers of persons who could learn esophageal speech. Stern (728) reported that, of over one hundred patients, only two failed to develop pseudovoice. Typical of statements in the 1930's and 1940's were "almost everyone can learn" or "those who really desire to learn."

More recent and realistic studies indicate that from 12 to 33 per cent of those surveyed could not or did not develop esophageal speech. The latest survey of the American Cancer Society states that 69 per cent of laryngectomees use esophageal speech. Were good instruction always available, then Greene's (277) figure of 80 per cent appears reasonable.

Along with overoptimism for the development of esophageal speech, there developed an unwarranted critical attitude toward the artificial larynx. Greater tolerance, understanding, and publicity might well have eased the way for those reluctant to use this aid.

Among those who cannot or should not develop esophageal speech are the following:

1.   The aged, who have often long since retired, may lack motivation and strength to learn to speak again. Recently the writer was asked to help an eighty-year-old American-Mexican whose only language was Spanish and who had received no information about esophageal speech or an artificial larynx. His speech needs were simple but of considerable personal importance. He desired to talk to some of his old cronies over a glass of beer, and he wanted to talk to his grandchildren in Spanish to keep the language alive in his family. The writer, speaking in the patient's native tongue, discussed the matter, played recordings, and demonstrated esophageal speech and the use of the artificial

larynx. The old man immediately decided on the artificial larynx, used it effectively, and has shown genuine gratitude for the assistance he received. No doubt many other elderly people should be dealt with in a similar manner.

2.   There are a few relatively young people who by reason of physical or psychological weakness may find it impractical to learn esophageal speech which is, after all, hard work unless one might use the "plosive" method exclusively—and the author doubts if this is possible. One of the author's patients is both physically and psychologically weak. She speaks with a buccal whisper which cannot be heard by the elderly relatives with whom she resides. We have given up trying to learn esophageal speech. The artificial larynx may be a crutch and a very useful one. Those who suffer a severe mental depression may be encouraged and helped by an artificial larynx.

3.   In some cases, physical structure or specific function precludes pseudovoice. By way of example, one must consider (a) destruction of tissue, (b) stenosis of the esophagus, (c) suspected recurrence of disease, (d) deafness on the part of the laryngectomee, his spouse, or other close companions.

4.   Occasionally one meets an individual who has little need for speech and for whom an artificial larynx supplies certain basic speech needs. The writer worked with a forty-five-year-old janitor whose first question in the hospital was, "Can I keep on drinking?" There was no serious question about learning speech. Now and then, for a social weekend, he would borrow an artificial larynx from an acquaintance.

The first artificial larynx was, insofar as we can determine, conceived by Czermak and executed by Brucke (380) in 1859, fourteen years before the first laryngectomy and approximately eighteen years after Reynaud (619) reported what may be the first case of esophageal speech. Czermak's patient presented complete laryngeal stenosis. The instrument was actuated by a reed and driven from the tracheal stoma. Although the prototype of all artificial vibrators, it was not highly successful.

In 1873, Billroth (380) in Vienna accomplished the first successful total extirpation of the larynx. His patient was fitted with an artificial larynx which was unique in its complexity, for it consisted of three parts: a tracheal, a pharyngeal, and a phonation cannula. The complexity of the instrument was no doubt "justified" by the fact that the operation of that day left a pharyngeal opening.

Complex instruments were no longer in order after Gluck's (17) modification of the laryngectomy which introduced closure and attachment of the tracheal tube to the skin of the neck. The food passage was now separate from the breathing passage, and food inhalation became impossible.

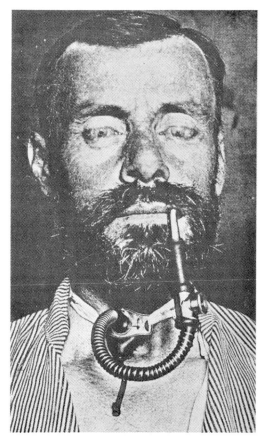

FIGURE 42. Gottstein's reed larynx in use in 1900. An inflatable rubber cushion sealed the tracheal tube. From Arnold (17).

It is interesting to note that, in 1873, Albert Billroth was a professor of surgery at Vienna, and that he had as a contemporary Herman Helmholtz, surgeon and physicist, who was then a professor of physics in Berlin. If Helmholtz had worked with Billroth, his acoustic sophistication and medical knowledge might well have led to the prompt development of an effective artificial larynx. As it was, Helmholtz was interested in the artificial larynx, but primarily because its operation supported his vowel theory.

The present author first had contact with an artificial larynx, and it was the reed type, in St. Louis in 1936 in the hands and mouth of a retired policeman. In originality it rivaled Billroth's and had been designed by its maker and user. The source of power was the hand-squeezed bulb of an old automobile horn of the type that once graced the side of a Stutz Bearcat. A tube led into the mouth where a re-formed clarinet reed vibrated with ample power and complexity.

The reed instrument is best represented by the Western Electric larynx developed in 1926, which is powered by breath from the tracheal stoma and which terminates in a reed held within the mouth. This instrument in the hands of a skilled operator gives good intelligibility and, according to a study by Hyman (343), is more pleasing to many ears than is esophageal speech. There are two major disadvantages : (1) The instrument is bulky and, with its loop of tubing from neck to mouth, presents a strange appearance. (2) Unless carefully and regularly cleaned, unpleasant odors develop. The Western Electric® reed instrument is superseded by the new W. E. 5a and 5b which will be discussed later. It is noted, parenthetically, that the Japanese have developed a very simple version of the reed larynx which retails for six dollars and fifty cents. It is easy to clean and renew, that is, the "reed" consists of a piece of rubber dam which can be cut from a large supply furnished with the instrument. The tone is loud and clear.

The Cooper-Rand Electronic Speech Aid® is the modern descendant of the first air-driven larynx, for it too pipes vibrations directly to the inside of the mouth. Manufactured by the Rand Development Corporation, this instrument is pictured in Figure

43. It consists of two elements; the first is a battery-powered transistorized oscillator which electronically generates the frequencies normally supplied by the vocal chords. The second element is the tone generator which is connected to the power supply by a fine wire. This tone generator takes the electric signal supplied by the oscillator and turns it into sound. This sound is directed into the mouth through a small plastic tube. Normal articulation of the lips and tongue turns these frequencies into intelligible speech."

The Cooper-Rand aid gives reasonable intelligibility and has a minimum amount of extraneous rattle; but one must learn to dodge the end of the transducer tube with the tongue, or speech

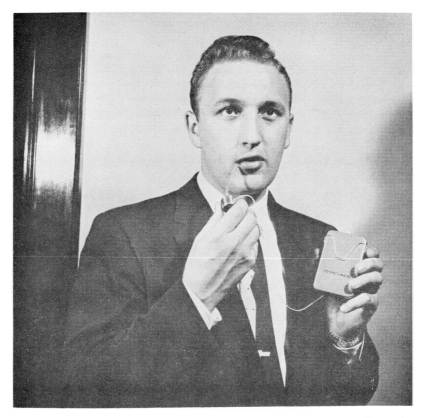

FIGURE 43. Cooper-Rand Electronic Speech Aid®. The energy from the transistor-actuated vibrator is transmitted by a small plastic tube to the inside of the mouth.

will be immediately and completely interrupted. Volume and pitch are adjustable. The intrument may be obtained encased in a smoking pipe.

Another type of aid which also vibrates directly in the mouth is the Oral Vibrator® developed by R. V. Tait, Rickmansworth, Herts, England. It is pictured in Figure 44.

> An upper dental prosthesis containing an electromagnetically vibrated diaphragm is incorporated in an artificial palate. The dental plate is connected by a fine twin-flex wire leading out of the mouth to a small battery-operated audio-oscillator, comparable in size to a hearing-aid and usually worn in a pocket. The dental appliance is constructed as an upper denture for patients who normally wear one, or may be held in position by the natural teeth in cases where no upper denture is worn.
>
> By pressing a small swith on the audio-oscillator, the diaphragm in the mouth is caused to vibrate. The sound produced in this way may be modulated into speech by normal speech-movements of the oral musculature. The oscillator is provided with a control whereby variations in pitch of voice may be obtained. The flex is detachable from the dental plate so that it need only be connected when the patient wishes to speak and is readily replaceable should breakage occur.

It should be remembered that many patients by the time cancer develops will have already been fitted with dentures. The instrument has very good intelligibility and a minimum of extraneous noise. All in all, the Oral Vibrator is relatively inconspicuous and a very promising development, but some would object to the wire that dangles from the mouth just as they might object to the wire and tube used with the Cooper-Rand Aid. For those who question the newness of almost everything, we should note that Gluck (17) experimented as early as 1914 with an instrument similar to Tait's vibrator.

The throat vibrator aids, as pictured in Figures 45 and 46, are modern versions of the oldest type of electrical aid. A pulsating disc sets the tissues of the throat vibrating. This type of aid is simple and rugged, but even the newest and best of them are somewhat noisy, though intelligible. The author did a paired-comparison study and found that superior esophageal speech was very much favored over speech from this type of artificial larynx.

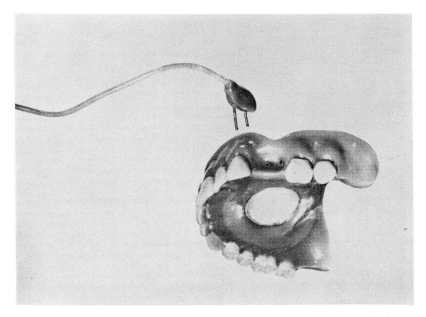

FIGURE 44. Tait's Oral Vibrator® (England). Like the Cooper-Rand, intra-oral vibration is utilized.

This is in contrast to Hyman's findings which favored the reed-type larynx.

Greene and Wright (17), in the early 1940's introduced the first workable electrolarynx which has subsequently been manu-factured and distributed widely through such companies as the Aurex Corporation. The Aurex® larynx has been continually im-proved and is highly favored by many laryngectomees.

The Kett, Mark III,® pictured in Figure 46 is especially to be recommended when the larynx is to be used under conditions of noise or when a laryngectomee is talking with someone who has marginal hearing. It is a powerful instrument that also has the advantage of being rechargeable. On the heavy side it should nevertheless be considered when conditions demand a relatively loud and intelligible instrument.

The Western Electric Electronic Larynx® throat vibrator is pictured in Figure 45. It is transistorized which makes for light-

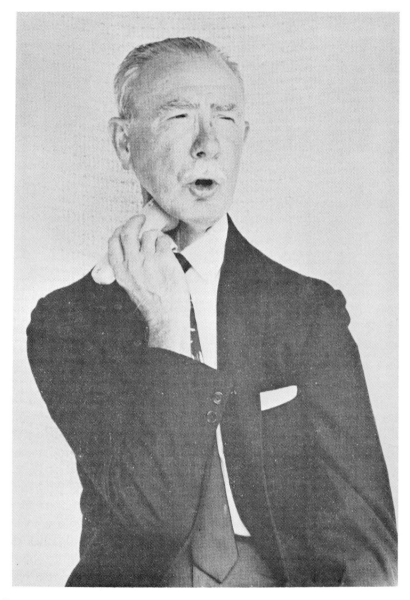

FIGURE 45. Western Electric (Bell Telephone) Electronic Larynx® with transistor vibrator.

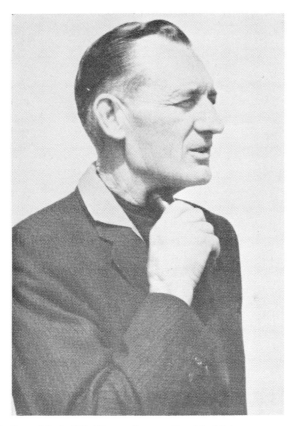

FIGURE 46. Kett Mark III Electro-Larynx® with high energy output. Self-contained batteries can be re-charged.

weight and economical utilization of batteries. The author noted the lack of loudness of this instrument, but it is inexpensive and has manual and continuous control of pitch modulation which serves to give some simulation of the complex changes in pitch found in the normal voice. The 5a model is pitched for the male voice, and the 5b for the female voice. The company states that intelligibility has been checked and found to be satisfactory. The Western Electric Model 5® supersedes the reed instrument which will no longer be manufactured but spare parts will remain available.

Speech Therapy

The acquisition of an artificial larynx gives little promise that clear and intelligible speech will automatically result because (1) The instrument is at best a crude vibrator, and the user must learn to articulate vowels clearly and with considerable exaggeration of mouth and tongue position. (2) Without support from pulmonary air, the consonants must be made in large part with buccal air. This new mode of articulation requires practice. (3) The larynx must be placed for optimum loudness. The location will vary from one subject to another. (4) Phrasing must be learned, that is, the larynx must be switched off at the end of phrases so that reasonably natural speech results. (5) A moderate rate of speech gives the best combination of efficiency and intelligibility. Trials at different rates will probably indicate that 150 words per minute should not be exceeded.

When one reviews the complexities of speech with the artificial larynx, it becomes evident that speech therapy will accelerate and refine the process of relearning speech. The efforts of the speaker and therapists are, however, much less arduous than is the case with esophageal speech. The exercises presented for esophageal speakers with especial reference to vowel, diphthong, and consonant drills will be found useful. If additional drill materials are needed, then a book containing these should be available. Fairbank's *Voice and Articulation Drillbook* is among those recommended.

Bibliography and References

JOHN O. ANDERSON AND JOHN C. SNIDECOR

T HE BIBLIOGRAPHICAL MATERIAL was gathered from many
sources. The major objective was to gather references, make
them as complete as possible, and standardize them with respect
to appropriate abbreviation.

The abbreviations adopted were from the publication *World
Medical Periodicals.* The first edition was prepared by a committee which was sponsored jointly by the United Nations Educational, Scientific, and Cultural Organization and the World
Health Organization. It was published in 1953. The second edition was prepared by L. T. Morton under the auspices of a committee jointly sponsored by the World Medical Association and
the International Union of the Medical Press and was published
in 1957. Where journals were not listed in either of the editions,
the articles in question were abbreviated in accordance with the
same principles of abbreviation, listed in the same form as found
in their published source, or written out in their entirety. The
basis for decision was clarity of reference.

Some bibliographical sources contained items for which incomplete listings were used. Usually these listings referred to
older publications or those not as widely circulated or utilized
as the major periodicals. When research utilizing the *Current List
of Medical Literature, Excerpta Medica, Index Medicus, the
Quarterly Cumulative Index Medicus,* and other standard bibliographical tools used for verification purposes failed to provide
complete information, entries were included in their incomplete
form. It was felt that this was preferable to omission.

The 1968 revision of the Bibliography and References was
completed by the senior author of the book. Over three hundred
items were added to those in the 1962 edition. It is hoped that
this bibliography will provide an accurate and useful tool to all
who are in need of this type of information.

1. ADAMS, M. R.: Communication aids for patients with amyotrophic lateral sclerosis. *J Speech Hearing Dis, 31:*274-75, 1966.
2. AGNELLO, J. G.: A Study of Intra- and Interphrasal Pauses and Their Relationship to the Rate of Speech. Unpublished Ph.D. dissertation, Ohio State University, 1963.
3. ALLEN: Faculte de parler sans larynx. *Med News (N. Y.),* March 17, 1894.
4. ALONSO, JUST M.: Conservative surgery of cancer of the larynx. *Trans Amer Acad Ophthal Otolaryng, 51:*633-42, July 1947.
5. ALVES, GARCIA: *Les Troubles du Langage.* Paris, Masson, 1951.
6. American Cancer Society, Inc.: Members of the American Speech and Hearing Association available for referral of laryngectomees. *Ca, 14:* 168-76, 1964.
7. American Cancer Society, Florida Division: *Your Latest Challenge, That New Voice.* 1964.
8. AMSTER, WALTER: A Comparative Study of the Breathing and Speech Coordination of Laryngectomized and Normal Subjects, and the Relationships Between the Breathing and Speech Coordinations and Articulatory Errors of Laryngectomized Subjects to Their Speech Intelligibility. Unpublished Ph.D. dissertation, Syracuse University, 1954.
9. ANDERSON, J. O.: Bibliography on esophageal speech. *J Speech Hearing Dis, 19:*70-72, 1954.
10. ANDERSON, J. O.: A Descriptive Study of Elements of Esophageal Speech. Unpublished Ph.D. dissertation, Ohio State University, 1950.
11. Anon.: Marine speaks again. *Time,* vol. 89, 1967.
12. Anon.: Finding his voice again. *Newsweek, 69:*86, 1967.
13. APPAIX, A.; STRIGLIONI, L., and DOR, A. M.: Bilan de la rééducation de 393 laryngectomisés—note technique. (Inventory of the vocal reeducation of 393 laryngectomees—technical note.) *J Franc Otorhinolaryng, 15:*419-26, 1966.
14. ARDISSONE: Causas de dificultad en la reeducacion de un laringectomizado. *Bol Soc Argentia de Logop y Foniatria,* vol. 6, 1951.
15. ARDRAN, G. M., and KEMP, F. H.: The mechanism of swallowing. *Proc Roy Soc Med, 44:*1038-40, 1951.
16. ARDRAN, G. M., and KEMP, F. H.: The protection of the laryngeal airway during swallowing. *Brit J Radiol, 25:*406-16, 1952.
17. ARNOLD, G. E.: Alleviation of alaryngeal aphonia with the modern artificial larynx. I. Evolution of artificial speech aids and their value for rehabilitation. *Logos, 3:*55-67, 1960.
18. Artificial larynx. *Pfizer Spectrum, 5:*439, 1957.
19. AVITABILLE, G.: La parotite post. operatoria. (Post-operative parotitis.) *Arch Ital Laring, 69:*655-59, 1961.
20. BABE, J., and DELGRADO, Y.: Technique personnelle de laryngectomie. *Rev Laryng (Bordeaux), 79:*577-80, 1958.

21. BACCARANI, O.: Respiratory tract of laryngectomized individuals: clinical and symptomatic study. *Otorinolarying ital*, vol. 12, 1942.

22. BADCOCK, M.: Speech therapy for certain vocal disorders. *J Laryng, 57:* 101, 1942.

23. BAILEY, BYRON J.: Partial laryngectomy and laryngoplasty: a technique and review. *Trans Amer Acad Ophthal Otolaryng, 70:*559-74, July 1966.

24. BAKER, H. K., and McDONALD, E.: Rehabilitation of the laryngectomized. *Crippled Child, 23:*10-11, 1950.

25. BALSHI, S.: Myoblastoma of the larynx. *Ann Otol, 69:*115-20, 1960.

26. BANDLER, A.: Ueber die Sprachbildung bei luftdichtem Kehlkopfverschlusse. *Z Heilk (Praha), 9:*423-32, 1888.

27. BÁNFAI, I.: Anatomische Rekonstruktion des Kehlkopfs nach horizontaler Resektion. (Anatomic reconstruction of the larynx after horizontal resection.) *Ann Laryng Rhinol Otol, 42:*32-38, 1963.

28. BANGS, J. L.: Bibliography on esophageal speech. *J Speech Dis, 12:*339-41, 1947.

29. BANGS, J. L.; BIERLE, D., and STROTHER, C.: Speech after laryngectomy. *J Speech Dis, 2:*171-76, 1946.

30. BARDIER, J.: La voix sans larynx. *Ann Otolaryng (Paris), 60:*131, 1943.

31. BARNEY, H. L.: Unitary transistorized artificial larynx. *IRE Wescon Convention Record,* part 8, p. 26, 1959.

32. BARNEY, H. L.: A discussion of some technical aspects of speech aids for post-laryngectomized patients. *Trans Amer Laryng Ass, 79:*103-15, 1958.

33. BARNEY, H. L.: The new Western Electric No. 5 type artificial larynx. *Logos, 3:*68-72, 1960.

34. BARNEY, H. L.; HAWORTH, F. E., and DUNN, H. K.: An experimental transistorized artificial larynx. *Bell System Tech J, 38:*1337, 1959.

35. BARROILHET, J.; FRENK, S., and HOLMGREN, B.: Vocal chord vibrations and EMG recorded in man after partial laryngectomy. *Pract Otorhinolaryng (Basel), 22:*244-47, 1960.

36. BARTALENA, G.: Certain olfactory secretory reflexes considered as the expression of olfactory capacity in laryngectomized. *Otorinolaring Ital, 20:*256-63, 1952.

37. BARTON, J., and HEJNA, R.: A Study of Factors Relating to Success or Non-success In the Acquisition of Esophageal Speech. Unpublished Seminar Report, Northwestern University, 1952.

38. BARTON, J., and HEJNA, R.: Factors associated with success or non-success in acquisition of esophageal speech. *J Speech Hearing Ass (Virginia), 4:*19-20, 1963.

39. BARTON, R. T.: Treatment of carcinoma of the larynx in the geriatric patient. *Geriatrics, 18:*283-90, 1963.

40. BARTON, R. T.: Life after laryngectomy. *Laryngoscope, 75:*1408-15, 1965.

41. BARTUAL, R.: Contribution a la technique de laryngectomie horizontale susglottique. (Contribution to the technique of supra-glottic horizontal laryngectomy.) *Rev Laryng Otol Rhinol, 83*:543-56, 1962.

42. BATEMAN, G. H.; DORNHORST, A. C., and LEATHHART, G. L.: Oesophageal speech. *Brit Med J, 2*:1177-8, 1952.

43. BATEMAN, G. H., and NEGUS, V. E.: Speech after laryngectomy. *Brit Surg Progr,* 1954, p. 105.

44. BATSON, O. V.: The cricopharyngeous muscle. *Ann Otol, 64*:47-54, 1955.

45. BAUTISTA, A. G.: Reconstruction following head and neck surgery and vocal rehabilitation of the laryngectomized. *Phillipp J Surg, 13*: 387-93, 1958.

46. BEATTY, H. C.: Cancer of the larynx and nasal accessory sinuses. *Ohio Med J, 43*:843-46, 1937.

47. BECK, J.: Living laryngectomized patients. *Arch Otolaryng (Chicago), 29*: 590, 1939.

48. BECK, J.: Phonetical examinations in laryngectomized. *Arch Ohr, Nas, Kehlkophfheilk, 165*:576-81, 1954.

49. BECK, J.: Substitute esophageal voice in laryngectomized. *Rev Laryng (Bordeaux), 77*:729-39, 1956.

50. BECK, J.: Zur Phonetik der Stimme u. Sprache Laryngektomierter. *Z Laryng Rhinol, 21*:506-21, 1931.

51. BECK, J. C., and POLLOCK, H. L.: Laryngectomy and laryngectomy case exhibition. *Ann Otol (St. Louis), 34*:1265, 1925.

52. BECKETT, J. M., and HARPMAN, F. A.: Voice rehabilitation after laryngo-hypo-pharyngo-cervical oesophagectomy. *Med Press, 242*:156-59, 1959.

53. BECKMANN, G.: Correlation of the size and form of the air chamber and the quality of speech in laryngectomized patients. *Z. Hals-, Nas u Ohrenheilk., 4*:258-60, 1954.

54. BECKMANN, G.: Reeducation of the voice following laryngectomy. *Dtsch Med Wschr, 4*:357-58, 1953.

55. Bell Laboratories: New artificial larynx. *Trans Amer Acad Ophthal Otolaryng, 63*:548, 1959.

56. Bell Telephone Co.: *High Speed Motion Pictures of the Human Vocal Cords.* New York, Bell Telephone Laboratories, pp. 1-17. (Mimeographed lecture which accompanies film with the same title.)

57. BELLUSSI, G.: Il Problema della reintegrazione vocale negli esiti degli interventi sulla larynge e sulla farynge. *Atti Clinica O.R.L. (Torino), 8*:177, 1949.

58. BELLUSSI, G.: Phonetic problems following surgery of laryngeal cancer; radiographic, stroboscopic and oscillographic studies. *Minerva Otorinolaring, 2*:501-5, 1952.

59. BERG, J. VAN DEN: Functional study of the esophageal sphincter in relation to the esophageal voice. *Ann Otolaryng (Paris), 74*:411-13, 1957.

60. BERG, J. VAN DEN: The properties of the vocal cavities. *Folia phoniat (Basel), 6*:8-14, 1954.

61. BERG, J. VAN DEN: Roentgen film of esophageal speech. *Arch Ohr, Nas, Kehlkophfheilk, 169*:481-83, 1956.

62. BERG, J. VAN DEN, and MOOLENAAR-BIJL, A. J.: Crico-pharyngeal sphincter, pitch, intensity and fluency in oesophageal speech. *Pract Otorhinolaryng (Basel), 21*:298-315, 1959.

63. BERG, J. VAN DEN; MOOLENAAR-BIJL, A. J., and DAMSTÉ, P. H. :Oesophageal speech. *Folia Phoniat (Basel), 10*:2:65-84, 1958.

64. BERG, J. VAN DEN; ZANTEMA, J. T., and DOORNENBAL, P., JR.: On the air resistance and the Bernouilli effect of the human larynx. *J Acoust Soc Amer, 29*:626-31, 1957.

65. BERGER, F.: Über somatische Beschwerden nach Laryngektomie. (Somatic difficulties after laryngectomy.) *Z Laryng Rhinol Otol, 39*:499-504, 1960.

66. BERGER, W.: 'Beiträge zur Analyse pathologischer Stimmklänge. *Ber V Versamml Dtsch Ges F Spr U Stimmhlk (Berlin)*, 1936.

67. BERGER, W.: Ueber subglottische Druckmessung bei Kanülenträgen. *Z Laryng usw, 25*:28, 1934.

68. BERING, L. H.: Om strubekraefter og dens behandling. *Tale og Stemme, 7*:1-13, 1943.

69. BERLIN, C. I.: Clinical measurement of esophageal speech. I. Methodology and curves of skill acquisition. *J Speech Hearing Dis, 28*:42-51, 1963.

70. BERLIN, C. I.: Clinical measurement of esophageal speech. III. Performance of nonbiased groups. *J Speech Hearing Dis, 30*:174-83, 1965.

71. BERLIN, C. I.: Hearing loss, palatal function, and other factors in postlaryngectomy rehabilitation. *J Chronic Dis, 17*:677-84, 1964.

72. BERLIN, C. I., and ZOBELL, D. H.: Clinical measurement during the acquisition of esophageal speech. II. An unexpected dividend. *J Speech Hearing Dis, 28*:389-92, 1963.

73. BERNHARDSGRUTTER, O.; LOHR, B., and SCHWAB, W.: Spirometric and bronchospirometric studies in laryngectomized patients. *Arch Ohr, Nas, Kehlkophfheilk, 166*:476-86, 1955.

74. BERNSTEIN, L., and HOLT, G. P.: Correction of vocal cord obduction in unilateral recurrent laryngeal nerve paralysis by transposition of the sternohyoid muscle. *Laryngoscope, 77*:876-85, 1967.

75. BILLROTH, C. T. (DR. CARL GUSSENBAUER, Asst. to Prof. Billroth): Ueber die erste druch Th. Billroth am Menschen. Ausgefuhrte Kehlkepf-Extirpation und die Anwendung Eines kuntstlichen Kahlkopfes. *Arch Klin Chir, 17*:343-56, 1874.

76. BIRD, H. M.: The speaking-aid. *Lancet, 1*:813-14, 1965.

77. BISI, R. H., and CONLEY, J. J.: Psychologic factors influencing vocal rehabilitation of the postlaryngectomy patient. *Ann Otol, 74*:1073-78, 1965.

78. BLACK, J. W.: A study of voice merit. *QJS, 28*:67-74, 1942.

79. BLUEMLEIN, H., and SCHMIDT, H.: Die Geschlechtsdifferenz der Kehl-kopfund Lungen-Karzinome. (Sex differences in cancer of the larynx and lungs.) *Z Laryng Rhinol Otol, 40:*639-44, 1961.

80. BOCCA, E.: Evidement "Fonctionnel" du cou dans la thérapie de prin-cipe des metastases ganglionnaires du cancer du larynx ("Func-tional" currettage as the fundamental treatment of ganglionic metastases of cancer of the larynx.) *J Franc Otorinolaryng, 13:*721-23, 1964.

81. BOHME, G., and SCHNEIDER, H. G.: Die Pathophysiologie des Laryngek-tomierten im Zusammenhang mit der Güte der Sprechfunktion. (The pathophysiology of the person without larynx in regard to the quality of his speech.) *Z Laryng Rhinol Otol, 39:*512-20, 1960.

82. BONDARENKO, E. D.: Raxvitie xvuchnoi rechi u bol'nykh posle laringek-tomii. (Development of voiced speech in patients after laryngectomy.) *Vestn Otorinolaring, 24:*77-79, 1962.

83. BOSE, H.: *Die Verengerung und Verschliessung des Kehlkopfes.* Giessen, W. Keller, 1865.

84. BRANKEL, O.: Patho-Physiologie der Pseudosprache Laryngektomierter. *Arch Ohr, Nas, Kehlkopfheilk, 165:*570-76, 1954.

85. BRANKEL, O.: X-ray stroboscopy of the form and position of the pseudo-glottis after laryngectomy. *Folia Phoniat, (Basel), 9:*18-31, 1957.

86. BRAUERS, quoted by EHRMANN: *Histoire de Polypes du Larynx.* Stras-bourg, Berger-Levrault, 1850.

87. BRAUN: Totale Kahlkopfexstirpation. Sprache mit und ohne küenst-lichen kehlkopf. *Deutsch Med Wschr, 5:*118, 1901.

88. BRIANI, A. A.: *Metodo di plastica cutaneo faringea per protesi fonetica in laryngectomizzati.* Venezia, Tipografia Commerciale, 1946.

89. BRIANI, A. A.: Speech rehabilitation in laryngectomized by means of expired air. *Arch Ital Otol, 63* (suppl. 12) :469-75, 1952.

90. BRIGHTON, G. R., and BOONE, W. H.: Roentgenographic demonstration of method of speech in cases of complete laryngectomy. *Amer J Roentgen, 38:*571-83, 1937.

91. BRODNITZ, F. S.: *Vocal Rehabilitation.* Rochester, Whiting, 1959.

92. BRODNITZ, F. S.: Semantics of the voice. *J Speech Hearing Dis, 32:*325-30, 1967.

93. BROWN, R. G.: A simple but effective artificial larynx. *J Laryng, 40:*739, 1925.

94. BRUNETTI, F.: Nachforschungen über die Tätigkeit des Schlundes bei Patienten, die am Kelkopf operiert wurden. *Arch Ohr Nas Kehl-kopfheilk, 149:*491-96, 1941.

95. BRUNETTI, F., JR.: Observations of the respiratory dynamic in laryngec-tomized patients. *Acta Otolaryng (Stockholm), 50:*334-43, 1959.

96. BRUNNER, H.: X-ray examination of the crico-pharyngeal sphincter — "Hypopharyngeal bar." *J Laryng Otol, 66:*276-82, 1952.

97. BRUNNER, H.: Cricopharyngeal muscle under normal and pathological conditions. *Arch Otolaryng, 56:*616-34, 1952.

98. BRUNO, G.; PALUDETTI, G., and PARONI, F.: Radiographic findings on the localization of the pseudoglottis during the emission of the voice in the laryngectomized. *Clin Otorinolaring, 5:*329-40, 1953.

99. BRUNS, P.: Die Laryngotomie sur Entfernung intra-laryngealex Neubildungen. *Wien Med Pr,* Nov. 1878.

100. BRUNS, P.: Ueber einige Verbesserungen des Küenstlichen Kehlkopfes. *Arch Klin Chir., 26:*780-83, 1881; *Deutsch Ges Chir, 10:*Kongr. (Part II) 1881, p. 51.

101. BURGER, H.: Speech without a larynx. *J Laryng, 40:*789-92, 1925.

102. BURGER, H., and KAISER, L.: Speech after laryngectomy. *Nederl T Geneesk, 2:*906-17, 1925.

103. BURGER, H.: Speech without a larynx. *Acta Otolaryng (Stockholm), 8:* 90-116, 1925.

104. CABANA, R.: La rehabilitation oral del laringectomizado. *Rev Cuba Otorinolaring, 3:*138, 1954.

105. CALDERIN, A. M.: Scientific principles in surgery of laryngeal cancer. *An Acad Nac Med (Madrid), 67:*491-527, 1950.

106. CAMERON, C. S.: *The Truth About Cancer.* Englewood Cliffs, Prentice-Hall, 1956.

107. CAMERON, C. S.: We speak again. *Mod Med, 17:*69-70, 1949.

108. CAMPANELLI, P. A.: Audiologic considerations in achieving esophageal voice. *Eye Ear Nose Throat Monthly, 43:*76, 78, 80; 1964.

109. CAMPBELL, C. J., and MURTAGH, J. A.: The simulated larynx. *Ann Otol, 68:*372-92, 1959.

110. CASADESUS: Phonetic apparatus for laryngectomized. *An Acad Med Quir Esp, 10:*109, 1923.

111. CASADESUS, F.: Indications et resultats a cinq ans de la laryngectomie totale dans les tumeurs du larynx et de L'hypopharyns. (Indications and results of 5 years of total laryngectomy in tumor of the larynx and hypopharynx.) In Leroux-Robert, J. (Ed.): *Advances in Oto-Rhino-Laryngology.* Basel, S. Karger, vol. IX, pp. 163-92, 1961.

112. CASTELLINI, G.; FRANZONI, M., and ZARABINI, G. E.: Modificazioni funzionali e scintigrafiche della tiroide nella chirurgia laringea. (Functional and scintigraphic changes of the thyroid in laryngeal surgery.) *Minerva Otorinolaring, 15:*51-55.

113. CAULK, R. M.: Laryngeal cancer: end results of radiotherapy based on clinical staging by TNM system. *Amer J Roentgen, 96:*588-92, 1966.

114. CELESTINO, D., and CURI, L.: Rivievi statistici sulla mortalità per cancro laringeo in Italia dal 1881 al 1962. (Statistics on the mortality rate due to laryngeal cancer in Italy from 1881 to 1962.) *Clin Otorinolaring, 17:*329-41, 1965.

115. CERNOCH, Z., and ZBORIL, M.: Rentgenkinematograficke zaznamy Jic-

novereci. (Roentgen clinematographic records of esophageal speech.) *Cesk Roentgen, 15*:85-02, 1961.

116. CHAPIN, A. B.: New voices after laryngectomy. *Ohio Speech Hearing Therapist,* 2:1-2, 1949.

117. CHEN, L.-C. Y.; SAMBERG, H. H., and FELSENSTEIN, B.: Aspects of rehabilitation of the laryngectomized patient. *Arch Phys Med, 44:* 267-72, 1963.

118. CHILOFF, C. L.: Contribution a' l'étude du developement du langage chez les laryngectomises. *Rev Laryng (Bordeaux),* 1925, p. 581.

119. CIMINO, A., and BERNICCHI, L.: Rilievi di broncoscopia, broncografia e termometria tracheo-bronchiale nei soggetti laringectomizzati. (Observations of bronchoscopy, bronchography and tracheobronchial thermometry in patients submitted to laryngectomy.) *Valsalva, 36:* 319-35, 1960.

120. CIURLO, E., and OTTOBONI, A.: La voce alaringea dei laringectomizzati. (The alaryngeal voice of the laryngectomized.) *Minerva Otorinolaring, 10*:69-75, 1960.

121. CLEMINSON, F. T.: Method of increasing audibility of speech after laryngectomy. *Proc Roy Soc Med, 22.* Section 24, 1928-29.

122. CLERF, L. H., and PUTNEY, F. G.: Cricopharyngeal spasm. *Laryngoscope, 52*:944-53, 1942.

123. Cleveland Hearing and Speech Center: *New Voices.* A training film. 1948.

124. CLEVES, C.: Rehabilitacion de la voz despues de la laryngectomia total *Rev Fac Med (Bogotá) 18*:405, 1949.

125. COJAZZI, L.: Sulla funzione esofagea esonetica vicariante nei laringectomizzatti. *Atti Laborat Fonetica. Univ Padova, 1*:41, 1949.

126. COLE, WARREN H.: Laryngectomees live constantly in peril. *St. Louis, Mo. Globe-Democrat.* August 3, 1960.

127. CONLEY, J. J.: Psychologic factors in carcinoma of the head and neck. *J Int Coll Surg, 31*:201-14, 1959.

128. CONLEY, J. J.; DEAMESTI, F., and PIERCE, M. K.: A new surgical technique for the vocal rehabilitation of the laryngectomized patient. *Ann Otol, 67*:655-64, 1958.

129. COOPER, H. K., and MILLARD, R. T.: A dental approach to speech restoration in the laryngectomee. *Dent Dig, 65*:106-12, 1959.

130. COOPER, M., Personal and written communication, 1967.

131. Cordless speech. *Time, 73*:72-74, April 13, 1959.

132. CORNUT, G.; VALLERY, J., and RICHAUD, M. C.: L'avenir social des laryngectomisés. (The social future of the laryngectomised.) *J Franc Otorinolaring, 11*:653-56, 1962.

133. CORUZZI, C.: Medico social importance of reeducation in laryngectomy. *Minerva Med, 44*:1047-49, 1953.

134. COVA, P., and ANTONIAZZI, B.: Resultats statistiques de 313 cas de can-

cers du larynx traites par la roentgen-therapy de 1928 a' 1946 a' l'Institut National du Cancer de Milan. *Radiol Clin, 21:4,* 1952.

135. COWAN, M.: Pitch and intensity of characteristics of stage speech. *Arch Sp,* suppl., 1936.

136. CRACOVANER, A. J., and RUBENSTEIN, A. S.: Dilation of the pharyngo-esophagus following total laryngectomy. *Arch Otolaryng (Chicago), 62:*303-07, 1953.

137. CRAMER, I. I.: Heat and moisture exchange of respiratory mucous membrane. *Ann Otol, 66:*327, 1957.

138. CRILE, G. W.: Laryngectomy. *Surg Gynec Obstet, 34:*305-6, 1922.

139. CROUSE, GERTRUDE PAT: An Experimental Study of Esophageal and Artificial-larynx Speech. Unpublished master's thesis, Emory University, 1962.

140. CROWE, S. J., and BROYLES, E. H.: Carcinoma of the larynx and total laryngectomy. *Ann Otol, 47:*875, 1938.

141. CUNNING, D. S.: Diagnosis and treatment of laryngeal tumors. *JAMA, 142:*73, 1950.

142. CURRY, E. T., and SNIDECOR, J. C.: Physical measurement and pitch perception in esophageal speech. *Laryngoscope, 71* (4) :3-11, 1961.

143. CUTLER, MAX.: Radiotherapy of early cancer of the larynx, 5 year results in 156 cases. *JAMA, 142:*957-63, 1950.

144. CZERMAK, J.: Ueber die Sprache bei luftdichter Verschliessung des Kehlkopfs. *S B Akad Wiss Wien, 35:*65, 1859.

145. CZERNY, V.: Versuche ueber Kehlkopfexstirpation. *Wien Med Wschr, 20:*557, 591; 1870.

146. DAHM, M.: Schluckstörungen und Schlucklähmungen. *Fortschr Roentgenstr, 64:*167, 1941.

147. DAHMANN, H.: Ueber die Lumen -u. Druckverhältnisse in der Speiseröhre. *Z Hals Nas Ohrenheilk, 7:*329-77, 1924.

148. DALY, J. F.: Treatment of carcinoma of the extrinsic larynx and laryngopharynx. *New York J Med, 52:*23, 1952.

149. DAMSTÉ, P. H.: Improvement of the voice after total laryngectomy by changing the site of the pseudoglottis. *Pract Otorhinolaryng (Basel), 19:*309-12, 1957.

150. DAMSTÉ, P. H.: Oesophageal speech. *Nederl T Geneesk, 101:*1784-86, 1957.

151. DAMSTÉ, P. H.: *Oesophageal Speech After Laryngectomy.* Groningen, 1958.

152. DAMSTÉ, P. H.: The glosso-pharyngeal press. *Speech Path Ther, 2:*70-76, 1959.

153. DAMSTÉ, P. H.: The artificial larynx. *Pract Otorhinolaring (Basel), 25:* 120-21, 1963.

154. DAMSTÉ, P. H.: Revalidatie na laryngectomie. (Rehabilitation after laryngectomy.) *T Revalid, 11:*443-52, 1965.

155. DAMSTÉ, P. H.: Clubs for the laryngectomized. *Folia Phoniat (Basel), 17:* 76-79, 1965.

156. DAMSTÉ, P. H.: Rehabilitation after laryngectomy. *Rehab Lit, 27:*266-68, 1966.

157. DAMSTÉ, P. H.; BERG, J. VAN DEN, and MOOLENAAR-BIJL, A. J.: Intake of air in oesophageal speech. *Acta Physiol Pharmacol Neerl, 5:*238-9, 1956.

158. DAMSTÉ, P. H.; BERG, J. VAN DEN, and MOOLENAAR-BIJL, A. J.: Why are some patients unable to learn esophageal speech? *Ann Otol, 65:* 998-1005, 1956.

159. DARLEY, F. L.: A Normative Study of Oral Reading Rate. M.A. thesis, State University of Iowa, 1940.

160. DAVIS, HALLOWELL (Ed.) : *Hearing and Deafness.* New York, Rhinehart, 1947, p. 475.

161. DEBINA, T.: Przetoki gardowe jako powiklania w przebiegu pooperacyj-nym raka krtani. (Pharyngeal fistulas as a complication in the course of post-surgery cancer of the larynx.) Summary. *Otolaryng Pol, 19:*127-28, 1965.

162. DE BRUINE, GROENEVELDT: De spraak na estirpatie van het strottenhoofd. *Nederl T Geneesk, 68:*1148-49, 1924.

163. DECROIX, G., and DEPOORTER, R.: Voice without larynx; reeducation after laryngectomy. *Lille Chir, 7:*82-4, 1952.

164. DECROIX, G., and DEPOORTER, R.: The voice without a larynx. *Montpellier Med, 55:*246-52, 1959.

165. DECROIX, G.; LIBERSA, C., and LATTARD, R.: Bases anatomiques et physiologiques de la reeducation vocale des laryngectomises. (The anatomical and physiological foundations of voice reeducation in laryngectomees.) *J Franc Otolaryng, 7:*549-73, 1958.

166. DEJUAN, P.: A laryngeal voice. *Acta Otolaring Iber Amer, 8:*411-32, 1957.

167. DEL CAÑIZO SUAREZ, C.; PISON, E.; BLANCO, R. B.; CONSUEGRA, R.; MARTIN, J. E., and CASARES, F. L.: Los cánceres de la cuerda vocal. (Cancer of the vocal cords.) *Acta Otorhinolaryng Espan, 11:*5-8, 1960.

168. DE MENA, J. M.: Problems of the voice and speech: recommendations for training and reeducation. *Hisp Méd, 11:*315-22, 1954.

169. DÉNES, L.: Changed method of voice and speech after laryngectomy. *Orr Hetil, 82:*1237-38, 1938.

170. DEY, F. L., and KIRCHENER, J. A.: The upper esophageal sphincter after laryngectomy. *Laryngoscope, 71:*99-115, 1961.

171. DICARLO, L. M.; AMSTER, W., and HERRER, G.: *Speech After Laryngectomy.* Syracuse, Syracuse, 1955

172. DIEDRICH, W. M., and YOUNGSTROM, K.: A Cineradiographic Study of the Pseudoglottis in Laryngectomized Patients. ASHA Convention Report, 1960.

173. DIEDRICH, W. M., and YOUNGSTROM, K.: An investigation of speech after laryngectomy, Final Report Project 337, *OVR*, 1961.
174. DIEDRICH, W. M., and YOUNGSTROM, K.: *Alaryngeal Speech*. Springfield, Thomas, 1966, p. 220.
175. DiSIMONE, G.: Radiokymographic study of the esophagus in laryngectomized subjects. *Ann Radiol Diagn (Bologna), 28:*372-82, 1955.
176. DOEHLER, MARY: *Esophageal Speech*. Boston, Amer Cancer Society, 1953.
177. DOHLMAN, G., and MATTESON, O.: The role of the cricopharyngeal muscle in cases of hypopharyngeal diverticula. A cineroentgenographic study. *Amer J Roentgen, 81:*561-69, 1959.
178. DORNHORST, A. C., and NEGUS, V. E.: Speech after removal of upper end of esophagus and the larynx. *Brit Med J, 4878:*16-17, 1954.
179. DROST, H. A.: Das Sprechen nach Entfernung des Kehlkopfes. (Speech After Laryngectomy.) München, J. F. Lehmanns Verlag, 1965, pp. 12.
180. DRUMMOND, S.: The effects of environmental noise on pseudovoice after laryngectomy. *J Laryng Otol, 79:*193-202, 1965.
181. DRUMMOND, S.: Vocal rehabilitation after laryngectomy. *Brit J Dis Communica, 2:*39-44, 1967.
182. DUB, A.: Algunas Concideraciones Sobre el Languaje del Laringectomizado. Il Congreso Sub-Americano de O. R. L., 1944, p. 333.
183. DUB, A.: A method for the development of oesophageal voice by the laryngectomized. *An Fonol Audiol (B. Aires), 2:*6-12, 1956.
184. DUB, A.: Social centers for patients after larynx surgery (in Uraguay). *Arch Ohr Nas Kehlfopfheilk, 165:*568-70, 1954.
185. DUFOUR, A., and FELLETTI, V.: Studio laringografico dei pazienti sottoposti ad intervento di laringectomia orizzontale sopraglottica. (Laryngographic studies of patients with horizontal supraglottic laryngectomies.) *Arch Ital Otorhinolaryng, 75:*567-604, 1964.
186. DUGUAY, M. J.: Preoperative ideas of speech after laryngectomy. *Arch Otolaryng, 83:*237-40.
187. DUNN, H. K.: The calculation of vowel resonances and an electrical vocal tract. *J Acoust Soc Amer, 22:*740, 1950.
188. DUPUY, H.: Voice without larynx. *New Orleans Med Surg J, 82:*791-92, 1930.
189. Editorial: Artificial larynx. *Pfizer Spectrum, 5:*439, 1957.
190. Editorial: Pipa di Ticchioni. *Gazz Sanit (Milano).* 1955.
191. Editorial: Speech after laryngectomy. *Eye Ear Nose Throat Monthly, 19:* 373, 1941.
192. EHRLICH, N.: *The Life of a Laryngectomee.* New York, Froben, 1937.
193. EHRMANN, C. H.: *Historie de Polypes du Larynx.* Strasbourg, Berger-Lebrault, 1850.
194. EQUEN, M.: The rehabilitation of the laryngectomee. *Arch Otolaryng (Chicago), 64:*1-2, 1956.
195. ERBSLÖH, H.: Kehlkopfverletzungen. *Arch Sprach Stimmheilk.* 1937.

196. ERICH, J. B.: Partial cicatricial stenosis of the hypopharynx: report of a case. *Laryngoscope, 72*:886-91, 1962.

197. EWANOWSKI, S.: Total laryngectomy and alaryngeal voice rehabilitation: case history. *Wisconsin Med J, 65*:210-13, 1966.

198. FAABORG-ANDERSON, K.: Electromyographic investigations of intrinsic laryngeal muscles in humans. *Acta Physiol Scand, 41*, suppl. 140, 1957.

199. FABRICANT, N. E.: Esophageal speech. *Eye Ear Nose Throat Monthly, 32:* 98-104, 1953.

200. FAIRBANKS, G.: *Voice and Articulation Drillbook.* New York, Harper, 1959.

201. FALBE-HANSEN, J.: Om stubekraeften og dens behandling. *Tale og Stemme, 7*:57, 1943.

202. FALK, P.: Erfahrungen mit der Garcia-Hormaeck-Naht nach Totalext. des Kehlkopfes. *Z Laryng Rhinol, 35*:158, 1956.

203. FARINA: La voz vicariante en los laryngectomizados. *Rev Esp Amer Laryng Otol Rinol,* 1949, p. 33.

204. FATIN, M.: Total laryngectomy in Egypt. *J Egypt Med Ass, 38*:419-27, 1955.

205. FAULKNER, W. B.: Objective esophageal changes due to psychic factors; an esophagoscopic study with report of 13 cases. *Amer J Med Sci, 200*:796-803, 1940.

206. FERRARI, R. C.: Radiological modifications of the esophagus subsequent to esophageal phonation. *Bol Trab Acad argent cir, 35*:420-22, 1951.

207. FERRARI, R. G.: Sobre el mechanismo de la fonación esofagica después de la laringectomia. *Bol Inst Clin Quir (B. Aires), 23*:104, 1947.

208. FIGI, F. A.: Hemilaryngectomy with immediate skin graft for removal of cancer of the larynx. *Trans Amer Acad Ophthal Otolaryng, 58*:22, 1954.

209. FIORI-RATTI, L.; COLLATINA, S., and CATASTA, G. M.: Proposta di un nuovo metodo per la valutazione obiettiva del grado di rieducazione con voce esofagea dei soggetti laringectomizzati. (A new method for the objective evaluation of esophageal voice in laryngectomized patients.) *Valsalva, 41*:1-11, 1965.

210. FLANAGAN, J. L.: Estimates of intraglottal pressure during phonation. *J Speech Hearing Res, 2*:168-72, 1959.

211. FLATAU, TH.: Die Storungen der Stimme nach Lebensstufen und die Stimme der Kehlkopflosen. *Festschr Ino Kubo, Tokyo, Herald Press,* 1934, p. 41.

212. FLETCHER, H.: *Speech and Hearing in Communication.* New York, Van Nostrand, 1953.

213. FLETCHER, S. G.: Analysis of cinema films in diagnosis and research. *J Biol Photogr Ass, 26*:29-33, 1958.

214. FONTAINE, ANNE, and MITCHELL, JOYCE: Oesophageal voice: a factor of readiness. *J Laryng, 74*:870-76, 1960.

215. FORNASARI, G.: Considerations and research on olfactory functions in laryngectomy. *Boll Mal Orecch, 69*:27, 1951.

216. FORNS: Presentacion de Cilindros Fonograficos Impressionados por la Voz de un Laringectomizado. Il Congreso Espagonl O. R. L., Barcelona, 1899, p. 164.

217. FRANKE, P.: A Preliminary Study Validating the Measurement of Oral Reading Rate in Words Per Minute. M.A. thesis, State Univ. Iowa, 1939.

218. FRANKEL, B.: Ueuber den kuenstlichen Kehlkopf und die Pseudostimme. *Berl Klin Wschr, 31*:756, 1893.

219. FREUD, ESTI D.: Speech therapy: experience with patients who had undergone total laryngectomy. *Arch Otolaryng (Chicago), 48*:150-55, 1948.

220. FROESCHELS, E.: Ein Fall von Oesophagusatmung u. Oesophagusstimme nach Kehlkopfexpiration. *Wien Med Wschr, 78*:1435, 1928.

221. FROESCHELS, E.: Sprechen ohne Kehlkopf. *Wien Med Wschr, 64*:150, 1914.

222. FROESCHELS, E.: Therapy of the alaryngeal voice following laryngectomy; a contribution. *Arch Otolaryng (Chicago), 53*:77-82, 1951.

223. FROESCHELS, E.: *Twentieth Century Speech and Voice Correction*. Philadelphia, Philosophical Library, 1948.

224. FROESCHELS, E.: Über Oesophagusatmung eines Larynektomierten. *Wien Med Wschr, 76*:875, 1926.

225. FULLER, A. P.; FOZZARD, J. A., and WRIGHT, G. H.: Sphincteric action of cricopharyngeus; radiographic demonstration. *Brit J Ophthal, 32*: 32-35, 1959.

226. FUMAGALLI, G., and OTTOBONI, A.: Valutazione dei volumini polmonari 'statici' e 'dinamici' in soggetti portatori di neoplasia laringea. *Minerva Otorinolaring, 8*:57, 1958.

227. FUMEAUX, J.: La voix oesophagienne des laryngectomises. (Etude radio-cinematographique.) (The esophageal voice of laryngectomees. Radio-cinemagraphic study.) *Pract Otorhinolaryng (Basel), 23*:397-400, 1961.

228. GAILLARD, J.; CHARACHON, R.; LAPICOREY, G., and GUILLIEN, M.: Réticulosarcome du sinus piriforme. (Reticulosarcoma of the piriform sinus.) *J Franc Otorhinolaryng, 12*:715-18, 1963.

229. GAILLARD DE COLLOGNY, L.: Cancer simultane des deux cordes vocales. (Simultaneous cancer of the two vocal cords.) *J Franc Otorhinolaryng, 14*:331-38, 1965.

230. GARCIA-TAPIA, Y., and HERNANDO, R.: New process for the treatment of cancer of the larynx. *An Acad nac Med (Madrid), 67*:183-93, 1950.

231. GARDE, E.: Physiologie et pathologie de la voix oesophagienne. *Rev Laryng (Bordeaux)*, Supplement Février, 1953, p. 149.

232. GARDNER, W. H.: Adjustment problems of laryngectomized women. *Arch Otolaryng (Chicago), 83*:3142, 1966.

233. GARDNER, W. H.: Increasing need for training in esophageal speech. *ASHA, 4:*146-47, 1962.

234. GARDNER, W. H.: Laryngectomees, (neck breathers) in industry. *Arch Environ Health (Chicago), 9:*777-89, 1964.

235. GARDNER, W. H.: Laryngectomees in Ohio, *Ohio Med J, 58:*926-28, 1962.

236. GARDNER, W. H.: The laryngectomees organize. *Quart J Speech, 42:* 270, 1956.

237. GARDNER, W. H.: Problems of laryngectomees. *J Chron Dis, 13:*253-60, 1961.

238. GARDNER, W. H.: Rehabilitation after laryngectomy. *Public Health Nurs (New York), 43:*612-15, 1951.

239. GARDNER, W. H.: Rehabilitation program for laryngectomees, illustrated by four case reports. *Cleveland Clin Quart, 22:*70-5, 1955.

240. GARDNER, W. H.: Speech pathology. *Med Physics, 3:*637-41, 1960.

241. GARDNER, W. H.: Summary . . . Second Annual Institute on Voice Pathology, Presented by the Cleveland Hearing and Speech Center, August 10-15, 1953.

242. GARDNER, W. H.: The whistle technique in esophageal speech. *J Speech Hearing Dis, 27:*187-88, 1962.

243. GARDNER, W. H.: They will talk again. *Nurs Outlook, 2:*314-15, 1954.

244. GARDNER, W. H., and HARRIS, H. E.: Aids and devices for laryngectomees. *Arch Otolaryng (Chicago), 73:*145-52, 1961.

245. GARDNER, W. H.; HILL, S. D.: and CARANO, H. N.: Esophageal speech for a twelve-year-old boy. A case report. *J Speech Hearing Dis, 27:* 227-31, 1962.

246. GARIBAY, FERNANDEZ A.: Emotional aspects in the laryngectomized patient. *Cir Cir, 23:*575-85, 1955.

247. GATEWOOD, E. T.: Development of esophageal speech after laryngectomy. *Southern Med J, 36:*453-55, 1943.

248. GATEWOOD, E. T.: The mechanism of esophageal voice following laryngectomy. *Virginia Med Monthly, 71:*9-13, 1944.

249. GATEWOOD, E. T.: A simple and practical procedure for developing esophageal voice in the laryngectomized. *Ann Otol, 54:*322-27, 1945.

250. GATEWOOD, E. T.: A new and simple procedure for esophageal voice in the laryngectomized patient. *Virginia Med Monthly, 73:*206-09, 1946.

251. GEMELLI: La voce dei Laryngectomizzati rieducata. Symposium de Foniatria de Padua, 1951.

252. GENEREAUX, K. S., Letter and enclosure, June 3, 1967.

253. GIGNOUX, M.; MARTIN, H.; CAJGFINGER, H., and JACQUEMARD, C.: Prognostic des pharyngo-laryngectomies circulaires totales. (Prognosis for total circular pharyngo-laryngectomies.) *J Franc Otorhinolaryng, 15:*233-38, 1966.

254. GIGNOUX, M.; MARTIN, H., and CAMUSET, M.: A propos d'une tumeur

dite mixte du larynx. (Concerning a so-called mixed tumor of the larynx.) *J Franc Otorhinolaryng, 12:*679-81, 1963.

255. GILMORE, S. I.: Rehabilitation after laryngectomy. *Amer J Nurs, 61:* 87-89, 1961.

256. GILSE, P. H. G. VAN: Another method of speech without larynx. *Acta Otolaryng (Stockholm),* (suppl.) *78:*109-10, 1949.

257. GILSE, P. H. G. VAN: Early diagnosis of cancer of larynx. *Nederl T Geneesk, 93:*2122-27, 1949.

258. GILSE, P. H. G. VAN: Over perichondritis laryngea en de spraak zonder doorgankelijk strottenhoofd. *Nederl T Geneesk, 77:*2402, 1933.

259. GILSE, P. H. G. VAN: Über den Mechanismus des Ructus uws. *Arch Néerl Phon Exp, 5:*37, 1930.

260. GILSE, P. H. G. VAN: Various methods of substitution for human speech. *Nederl T Geneesk, 100:*453-58, 1956.

261. GIRAUD, J. C.; LEBON, P., and HADIDA, A.: De la fermeture des larges pharyngostomes apres laryngectomie pour cancer. (On the closure of large pharyngeal fistulas after laryngectomy for cancer.) *J Franc Otorhinolaryng, 10:*711-45, 1961.

262. GLASS, E. J. G., and FRASER, W. D.: Malignant disease involving the larynx in the elderly patient. *Geriatrics, 20:*228-35, 1965.

263. GLEITSMANN, J. W.: Laryngectomy: method of artificial voice production. *J Laryng, 24:*179-82, 1909.

264. GLUCK, TR.: Der gegenwaertige Stand der Chirurgie des Kehlkapfes, etc. *Mschr Ohrenheilk, 38:*141, 1904.

265. GLUCK, TR.: Die Chirurgie im Dienste der Layngologie. *Z Laryng Rhinol Otol, 1:*179, 1909.

266. GLUCK, TR.: Fluestersprache und phonationsapparate. *Berl Klin Wschr, 36:*215, 1899.

267. GLUCK, TR.: Patienten mit Total exstirpation des Pharynx, Larynx and Oesophagus denen eine kuenstliche Stimme durch automatisch arbeitenden Apparat geliefert wird. *Berl Klin Wschr, 47:*33, 1910.

268. GLUCK, TR.: Phonetik-Chirurgie der oberen Luft-und Speisewege und kuenstlicher oder natuerlicher Stimmersatz. *Mschr Ohrenheilk, 64:* 881, 1930.

269. GLUCK, TR.: Problems und Ziele der Chirurgie der oberen Luftwege. *Mschr Ohrenheilk, 55:*1150, 1921.

270. GLUCK, T., and SORENSEN, J.: *Die chirurgische Therapie des Kehlkopkarzinoms.* Jahresk. ärztl. Fortbild., München, 1912.

271. GÖBELL: Stimmbildung nach Kehlkopfextirpation. *Deutsch Med Wschr, 50:*1234, 1924.

272. GOETZINGER, C. P.; DIRKS, D., and BAER, C.: Auditory discrimination and visual perception in good and poor readers. *Ann Otol, 69:*121-26, 1960.

273. GOETZINGER, C. P.; PROUD, G. O.; DIRKS, D., and EMBREY, J.: A study of hearing in advanced age. *Arch Otolaryng (Chicago), 73:*662-74, 1961.

274. Goetzinger, C. P., and Rousey, C.: Hearing problems in later life. *Med Times, 87:*771-80, 1959.

275. Gottstein, G.: Pseudostimme nach Totalexstirpation des Larynx. *Arch Klin Chir, 62:*126-46, 1900.

276. Greene, J. S.: Composite postoperative therapy for the laryngectomized. *Laryngoscope, 53:*13-16, 1943.

277. Greene, J. S.: The postlaryngectomy clinic of the National Hospital for Speech Disorders; a statistical study of 300 patients. *New York J Med, 49:*2398-404, 1949.

278. Greene, J. S.: Rehabilitating the laryngectomized patient. *Bull Amer Cancer Soc, 24:*5, 1942.

279. Greene, J. S.: Speech rehabilitation following laryngectomy. *Amer J Nurs, 49:*413-31, 1949.

280. Greene, M. C. L.: Management of aphonia after surgical treatment of carcinoma of the larynx, pharynx and oesophagus. *Brit J Dis Communica, 2:*30-38, 1967.

281. Greiner, G. F.; Isch, F.; Isch-Treussard, C.; Ebtinger-Jouf-Froy, J.; Klotz, G., and Champy, M.: L'electromyographic appliquee a la pathologie du larynx. (Electromyography applied to the pathology of the larynx.) *Acta Otolaryng (Stockholm), 51:*319-31, 1960.

282. Grimaud, R., and Labaeye: Cancer du larynx et tuberculose pulmonaire. (Cancer of the larynx and pulmonary tuberculosis.) *J Franc Otorhinolaring, 14:*457-60, 1965.

283. Grimaud, R.; Pierson, B., and Wiadzalowski, G.: Papillomatose laryngée de l'enfance et dégénérescence maligne. (Laryngeal papillomatosis of childhood and malignant degeneration.) *J Franc Otorrinolaring, 10:*587-91, 1961.

284. Guerrier, Y., and Dejean, Y.: Apropos de onze observations de cancer du larynx. (On eleven observations of cancer of the larynx.) *J Franc Otorhinolaring, 12:*939-50, 1963.

285. Guns, P.: Laryngectomie reconstructive. *Rev Laryng (Bordeaux), 74:* 509-13, 1953.

286. Guns, P.: La voix après laryngectomie. *Rev Fr Phoniat, 1:*79, 1933.

287. Guns, P.: Production of voice after laryngectomy. *Scalpel (Brux), 86:*549-52, 1933.

288. Gussenbauer, C.: Ueber die erste durch Th. Billroth am Menschen ausgefuehrte Kehlkopf-Exstirpation under die Anwendung eines kuenstlichen Kehlkopfes. *Arch Klin Chir, 17:*343-56, 1874.

289. Guttman, M. R.: Rehabilitation of the voice in laryngectomized patients. *Arch Otolaryng (Chicago), 15:*478, 1932.

290. Guttman, M. R.: Tracheopharyngeal fistulization; a new procedure for speech production in the laryngectomized patient. *Trans Amer Laryng Rhinal Otol Soc, 41:*219-26, 1935.

291. Gutzmann, M.: Kann ein Patient ohne Kehlkopf wieder Sprechen? *Z Aerztl Fortbild (Jene), 30:*79, 1933.

292. GUTZMANN, M.: Sprache ohne Kehlkopf. *Deutsch Med Wschr, 60:*319, 1934.

293. GUTZMANN, M.: *Sprache ohne Kehlkopf.* Leipzig, C. Kabitsch, 1936.

294. GUTZMANN, H.: Stimme und Sprache ohne Kehlkopf. *Z Laryng Rhinol Otol, 1:*221, 1909.

295. GUTZMANN, H.: Über die Oesophagusstimme. *Deutsch Med Wschr, 13:* 520, 1925.

296. GUTZMANN, H.: Uber die Rehabilitation der Laryngektomierten. (Rehabilitation of the laryngectomee.) *Folia Phoniat, 14:*51-54, 1962.

297. GUYOT, C., and GUYOT, R. T.: Catalogue d'ètude dé ce qui a été publié jusqu'á nos jours sur les sourds-muets sur l'oreille, l'ouie, la voix, le langage, la mimique, les aveugles etc. Gronigen, 1842.

298. HAAGEN, C.: Intelligibility Measurement; Techniques and Procedures Used by the Voice Communications Laboratory. OSRD Report No. 5748, PB 121-69, May 1948.

299. HAASE, H.-J.: Psychologie und Psychopathologie Kehlkopfexstirpierter. Zur Bedeutung von Persönlichkeitsanlage, Erlebnis und Milieu. (Psychology und psychopathology after laryngectomy.) *Fortschr Neurol Psychiat, 28:*253-72, 1960.

300. HADWIGA, N.: Übungssystem zur Erlernung der Ersatzsprache nache Laryngektomie. (Systematic exercises for teaching pseudospeech after laryngectomy.) *HNO (Berlin), 8:*241-44, 1967.

301. HAJEK, M.: *Pathologie und Therapie der Erkrankungen des Kahlkopfes, der Luftröhre und der Bronchien.* Leipzig, Kabitsch, 1932.

302. HANDZEL, L., and GIERMANSKI, A.: Value of radiological investigations in vocal and speech rehabilitation following laryngectomy. *Pol Przegl Radiol, 23:*313-18, 1959.

303. HANLEY, C.; Unpublished case report.

304. HANLEY, T. D.: An analysis of vocal frequency and duration characteristics of selected samples of speech from three American dialects. *Sp Monog, 18:*78-93, 1951.

305. HANSON, H. V.: Carcinoma of the larynx, laryngectomy, artificial larynx. *Med Bull Veterans Adm (Wash.), 13:*61-3, 1936.

306. HANSON, W. L.: A new artificial larynx with a historical review. *Illinois Med J, 78:*483-86, 1940.

307. HARPMAN, J. A.: Cancer of the hypopharynx. *Eye Ear Nose Throat Monthly, 44:*51-54, 1965.

308. HARRIES, J. R., and LAWES, W. E.: The advantages of glossopharyngeal breathing. *Brit Med J, 2:*1204-5, 1957.

309. HARRINGTON, R.: Problems Associated with the Development of Pseudovoice in the Aged Laryngectomee. ASHA Convention Report, 1960.

310. HARROLD, C. C., JR.: The artificial pharyngeal pouch: another alternative in reconstruction after laryngectomy. *Cancer, 10:*928-32, 1957.

311. HARTENAU, W.: Die Sprechfunktion laryngektomierter. *Arch Ohr Nas Kehlkopfheilk, 156:*461, 1950.

312. HASS, W.: Die 'Sprechspange fur Kehlkopflose.' (A speech clasp for alaryngeal people.) *HNO (Berlin), 9:*26-27, 1960.

313. HAUTANT, A.: Hemilaryngectomie d'apres mon procédé. *Ann Mal Oreil Larynx,* May 1929.

314. HAUTANT, A., and OMBRÉDANNE, M.: Traitement chirurgical du cancer endolaryngé (L'hémi-laryngectomie). *Paris Méd, 1:*255-60, 1930.

315. HAWORTH, F. E.: An electronic artificial larynx. *Bell Lab Rec, 38:*362-68, 1960.

316. HEAVER, L., and ARNOLD, G. E.: Rehabilitation of alaryngeal aphonia. *Postgrad Med, 32:*11-17, 1962.

317. HEAVER, L.; WHITE, W., and GOLDSTEIN, N.: Clinical experience in restoring oral communication to 274 laryngectomized patients by esophageal voice. *J Amer Geriat Soc, 3:*687-90, 1955.

318. HENDRICK, J.: *Voice Without a Larynx.* Formal papers of American Society for Study of Speech. 1932. pp. 22-26.

319. HERNANDEZ, A.; SCHWARTZMAN, J.; RUZ, E., and SANCHEZ, E.: Phoniatric reeducation of laryngectomized patients. *Sem Med (B. Aires), III* (suppl. 15):748-49, 1957.

320. HERZOG, W., and NEUMANN, D.: Ein Künstlicher electronischer Kehlkopf. (An electronic artificial larynx.) *Phonetica, 13:*117-33, 1965.

321. HEYDEN, R.: The respiratory function in laryngectomized patients. *Acta Otolaryng (Stockholm),* (suppl.) *85.* 1950.

322. HINOJAR, A.: Simple Phonetic Apparatus. *An Acad Med Quir Esp, 10:* 93, 1923.

323. HJERPE, JOYCE A.: A Cineflurographic Study of Alaryngeal and Normal Speakers. Unpublished master's thesis, University of Kansas, 1962.

324. HOCHENEGG, J.: Totale Kehlkopfexstirpation etc., Ein neuer Sprechapparat. *Wien Klin Wschr, 5:*123, 1892.

325. HODSON, C. J., and OSWALD, M. V. O.: *Speech Recovery After Total Laryngectomy.* Baltimore, Williams & Wilkins, 1958.

326. HOFMANN-SAGUEZ, R.: La Laryngectomie reconstitutive. *Ann Otolaryng (Paris), 71:*405-15, 1954.

327. HOFMANN-SAGUEZ, R.: La laryngectomie reconstitutive; technique personelle; Presentation de film en couleurs. *Rev Laryng (Bordeaux), 74:*143-48, 1953.

328. HOLINGER, P. H. *et al.:* Cancer of the larynx. I. Surgical treatment. *Amer J Nurs, 57:*738-41, 1957.

329. HOMMERICH, K. W., and KUKLA, U.: Untersuchungen über den Spracherwerb nach Laryngektomie. (Investigation of speech acquisition following laryngectomy.) *Z Laryng Rhinol Otol, 44:*802-10, 1965.

330. HOOPLE, G. D., and BREWER, D. W.: Voice production in the laryngectomized patient. *Trans Amer Laryng Ass, 75:*155-67, 1954.

331. HOPMANN, E.: Stimmund Sprachstörungen nach Kehlkopfausrottung. *Deutsch Chir, 99:*301-5, 1909.

332. HORN, D.: *Laryngectomee Survey Report*. Eleventh Annual Meeting, International Association of Laryngectomees, Memphis, Tenn., August 21, 1962.

333. HOSHINO, T.: Complete extirpation of the larynx in carcinoma. *Ann Otol, 28:*466-72, 1919.

334. HOWIE, T. O.: Esophageal speech sounds as a means of intercommunication. *Surgo, 12:*14-19, 1945.

335. HOWIE, T. O.: Rehabilitation after total laryngectomy. *Glasg Med J, 27:* 45-8, 1946.

336. HOWIE, T. O.: Rehabilitation of the patient after laryngectomy. *Occup Ther, 26:*372-83, 1947.

337. HUDSON, A.: Communications problems of the geriatric patient. *J Speech Hearing Dis, 25:*238-48, 1960.

338. HUET, P. C., et NEMOURS-AUGUSTE: Etude radio-physiologique du premier temps de la déglutition, isolé. *Arch Mal Appar Dig, 32:*113, 167, 1943.

339. HUIZINGA, E.: Over de belangrijkheid van het aanzetstuk. *Log en Phon, 12:*718, 1940.

340. HUIZINGA, E.: Recherches sur un vertrilogue néerlandais. *Arch Neerl Phon Exp, 6:*1931.

341. HUIZINGA, E.: Kompensierung in Ansatzstück bei der Bildung von Selbstlauten. *Arch Neerl Phon Exp, 17:*1941.

342. HUNT, R. B.: Rehabilitation of the laryngectomee. *Laryngoscope, 74:* 382-95, 1964.

343. HYMAN, M.: An experimental study of artificial larynx and esophageal speech. *J Speech Hearing Dis, 20:*291-99, 1955.

344. HYMAN, M., and KELLER, M. S.: Como volver a habler. Amer Cancer Society, Ohio Division, 1966.

345. HYMAN, M., and KELLER, M. S.: *How to Speak Again.* A manual with a recording for laryngectomees. The Ohio Division of the American Cancer Society, 1960.

346. If you can burp, you will talk again. *Cancer Bull (Texas), 2:*130-31, 1950.

347. INGELFINGER, F. J.: Esophageal motility. *Physiol Rev, 38:*533-84, 1958.

348. IGLAUER, S.: Artificial larynx, with patient demonstrating its use. *Ann Otol, 45:*1176, 1936.

349. Institute on Voice Pathology. Proceedings first institute on voice pathology and the first international meeting of laryngectomized persons. Cleveland, Ohio. August 1-2, 1952.

350. Institute on Voice Pathology. Summary second annual institute of Pathology. Cleveland, Ohio. August 10-15, 1953.

351. International Association of Laryngectomees: *First Aid for Laryngectomees (Neck Breathers).* International Association of Laryngectomees, 219 East 42nd Street, New York, N. Y. 10017. 1962.

352. International Association of Laryngectomees: *Helping Words for the*

Laryngectomee. International Association of Laryngectomees, 219 East 42nd Street, New York, N. Y. 10017. 1964.

353. International Association of Laryngectomees: *Local Chapter Manual on Basic Organization and Program*. The International Association of Laryngectomees, 521 W. 57th Street, New York, N. Y.

354. INTRONA, F.: Retraining and rehabilitation of the laryngectomized as a medico-social problem. *Arch Ital Otol, 69*:228-37, 1958.

355. ISSHIKI, N.: Regulatory mechanism of voice intensity variation. *J Speech Hearing Res, 7*:17-29, 1964.

356. ISSHIKI, N., and SNIDECOR, J. C.: Air intake and usage in esophageal speech. *Acta Otolaryng, 59*:559-74, 1964.

357. ISSHIKI, N., and VON LEDEN, H.: Hoarseness-aerodynamic studies. *Arch Otolaryng (Chicago), 80*:206-13, 1964.

358. IWANOFF, A.: Ueber die stimme Laryngektomierter. *Z Laryng Rhinol (Würzb), 3*:131-38, 1910.

359. JACKSON, C.: les resultantes des methods operatoires dans le traitement du cancer du larynx. *Ann Mal Oreil Larynx, 41*:1221-39, 1922.

360. JACKSON, C. L.: Cancer of the larynx. *Postgrad Med, 6*:379, 1949.

361. JACKSON, C. L.: The voice after direct laryngoscopic operations, laryngo-fissure and laryngectomy. *Arch Otolaryng (Chicago), 31*:23-26, 1940.

362. JACKSON, C., and JACKSON, C. L.: *Diseases of the Nose, Throat and Ear.* Philadelphia, Saunders, 1946.

363. JACKSON, C., and JACKSON, C. L.: *The Larynx and Its Diseases.* Philadelphia, Saunders, 1937, pp. 408-09, 411.

364. JACKSON, C., and JACKSON, C. L.: Increasing incidence of cancer of the larynx. *Trans Amer Acad Ophthal Otolaryng, 45*:156-75, 1941.

365. JACKSON, C. L., and NORRIS, C. M.: Cancer of the larynx. Part II. Incidence and etiology — pathology and classification. *CA, 12*:56-62, 1962.

366. JACKSON, C. L., and NORRIS, C. M.: Indications and results after five years of total laryngectomy. In Leroux-Robert, J. (Ed.) : *Advances in Oto-Rhinol-Laryngology*. White Plains, Phiebig, 1961, Vol. IX, pp. 41-130.

367. JANOWSKI, W.; KANIOWSKI, T., and RECZEK, H.: X-ray picture of the hypopharynx in laryngectomized patients. *Pol Przegl Radjol, 23:* 15-18, 1959.

368. JEBURG, N.: Laryngectomy: past, present, and future. *Ann Otol, 69:* 184-98, 1960.

369. JESBURG, N.: Rehabilitation after laryngectomy. *Calif Med, 80*:80-82, 1954.

370. JESBURG, N.: Speech after laryngectomy. *Med Times, 84*:1312-14, 1956.

371. JIMENEZ: La Phonation chez un laryngectomisé. *Comptes Rendus de l'académ. Méd Chir espagnole*. April 14, 1921.

372. JIMISON, CARMIN: Cancer of the larynx. II. Nursing the patient after laryngectomy. *Amer J Nurs, 57*:741-43, 1957.

373. JOHANNESSEN, J. V., and FOY, A. L.: Team effort in the rehabilitation of laryngectomy patients. *J Amer Geriat Soc, 12:*1073-76, 1964.
374. JOHNSON, C. A.; HOLINGER, P., and ANDREWS, A.: Electrocardiogram changes after laryngectomy. *Arch Otolaryng (Chicago), 47:*835, 1948.
375. JOHNSON, C. L.: A survey of laryngectomee patients in Veteran's Administration hospitals. *Arch Otolaryng (Chicago), 72:*768-73, 1960.
376. JOURDAN, F., and COLLETT, A.: L'influence du pneumogastrique sur l'oesophage et l'estomac. *J Physiol (Paris), 41:*194A-95A, 1949.
377. KAISER, L.: Examen phonétique d'un sujet privé de larynx. *Arch Néerl Physiol, 10:*468, 1926.
378. KAISER, L., and BURGER, H.: Spraak zonder strottenhoofd. *Neder T Geneesk, 68:*2:906, 1925.
379. KALLEN, L. A.: Discussion of mechanism of esophageal speech. *Arch Otolaryng (Chicago), 15:*479, 1932.
380. KALLEN, L. A.: Vicarious vocal mechanisms: The anatomy, physiology and development of speech in laryngectomized persons. *Arch Otolaryng (Chicago), 20:*460-503, 1934.
381. KAMIETH, H.: Comparative x-ray investigation on esophageal speech in laryngectomized patient. *Radiol Clin. (Basel), 28:*88-101, 1959.
382. KAPLAN, S.: Zur Frage der Stimmgildung bei Laryngektomierten. Abstracted in *Zbl Hals Nas Ohrenheilk, 8:*716, 1926.
383. KATZ, B.: The IAL. *Cancer News, 14:*1:3-7, 1960.
384. KAUFMAN, H.: Carcinoma of larynx and hypopharynx: Telecaesium therapy. *Deutsch Med Wschr, 91:*339-45, 1966.
385. KELLEHER, W. H., and PARIDA, M. B.: Glossopharyngeal breathing. *Brit Med J, 2:*740-43, 1957.
286. KENESSEY, L.: The speech after laryngectomy. *Fulorrgegegyogyaszat, 2:* 79-83, 1957.
387. KINDLER, W.: Die Rehabilitation Kehlkopfloser nach Krebsausrottung. (Rehabilitation of laryngectomees after extirpation of cancer.) *Med Welt, 35:*1748-50, 1960.
388. KINDLER, W., and ULICH, H.: The olfactory capacity in laryngectomized and tracheotomized. *Arch Ohr Nas Kehlkopfheilk, 162:*512-19, 1953.
389. KING, H.: I lost my voice to cancer. *Sat Even Post,* Sept. 1, 1956.
390. KIRCHNER, J. A.; SCATLIFF, J. H., and SHEDD, D. P.: Cinefluorography in the pre- and postoperative management of laryngeal cancer. *Ann Otol, 69:*768-80, 1960.
391. KIRCHNER, J. A.; SCATLIFF, J. H.; DEY, F. L., and SHEDD, D. P.: The pharynx after laryngectomy. *Laryngoscope, 63:*18-33, 1963.
392. KLAJMAN, S., and BETLEJEWSKI, S.: Projekt klimatyzacj pomieszczenia dla laryngektomowanych. (A project of air conditioning for post laryngectomy individuals.) *Otolaryng Pol, 19:*28, 1965.
393. KLEINSASSER, O.: Kritische B trachtung der Behandlungsergebnisse bei 410 Kehlkopfkarzinomen unter besonderer Beruecksichtigung der

Indikation zur Radical Neck Dissection. (Critical consideration of results of treatment of 410 cases of carcinomata of the larynx with special regard to the indication for radical neck dissection.) *Z Laryng Rhinol Otol, 40:*652-74, 1961.

394. KLEINSASSER, O.: Über den krankheitsverlauf bei Epithelhyperplasien der Kehlkopfschleimhaut und die Entstehung vone Karzinomen. (Course of epithelial hyperplasias of the laryngeal mucosa and the formation of carcinomas.) *Z Laryng Rhinol Otol, 42:*541-58, 1964.

395. KLEINSASSER, O.: Über die Behandlung einfacher und präkanzeröser Epithelhyperplasien der Kehlkopfschleimhaut. (Treatment of simple and precancerous epithelial hyperplasia of the laryngeal mucosa.) *Z Laryng Rhinol Otol, 43:*14-24, 1964.

396. KLOPFER, F.: Speech education for laryngectomized subjects. *Orr Hetil, 91:*27, 1950.

397. KNEISNER, ERIKA: Exper. -phonetische Untersuchungen an einem Fall von willkürlicher Aerophagie. *Mschr Ohrenheilk, 66:*431, 1932.

398. KNEPFLAR, K.: Individualized Speech Therapy for Laryngectomized Patients. ASHA Convention Report, 1960.

399. KNEPFLAR, K.: Therapy approaches for the improvement and refinement of pseudovoice in laryngectomized speakers. *NZ Speech Therapist, 18:*18-22, 1963.

400. KOEPP-BAKER, H.: The rehabilitation of the laryngectomized. *Trans Amer Acad Ophthal Otolaryng, 52:*227-33, 1948.

401. KOEPP-BAKER, H., and McDONALD, E.: Rehabilitation of the laryngectomized. *Crippled Child, 30* (3) :10-11, 1950.

402. KOLSON, H., and GLASGOLD, A.: Tracheo-esophageal speech following laryngectomy. *Trans Amer Acad Ophthal Otolaryng, 71:*421-25, 1967.

403. KONEČNÝ, L.: Parciální operace laryngu pro karcinom. (Partial operations of the larynx for carcinoma.) *Cesk Otolarying, 9:*367-74, 1960.

404. KRAUSS: Formation artificelle de la parole aprés extirpation du larynx. *Allg Wien Med Zeitung, 19.* 1894.

405. KYTTA, J.: Finnish oesophageal speech after laryngectomy. Sound spectrographic and cineradiographic studies. *Acta Otolaryng (Stockholm),* suppl. 195, p. 94, 1964.

406. KYTTA, J.: Spectrographic studies of the sound quality of oesophageal speech. *Acta Otolaryng (Stockholm),* suppl. 188, 1964.

407. LAFON, J. C.: Etude acoustique de la voix oesophagienne. (Acoustical study of the esophageal voice.) *Rev Laryng (Bordeaux), 81:*271-80, 1960.

408. LAFON, J. C.: La notion d'impulsion et son application a l'etude de la structure de la voix et de la parole. (The concept of impulsion and its application to the study of the production of voice and of speech.) *J Franc Otorhinolaring, 11:*491-96, 1962.

409. LAFON, J. C., and CORNUT, G.: Acoustic study of the esophageal voice and verification of a structural identity with laryngeal voice. *C R Soc Biol (Paris), 152:*1535-37, 1958.

410. LAFON, C., and CORNUT, G.: Etude de la formation impulsionnelle de la voix et de la parole. (A study of the pulse production of voice and speech.) *Folia Phoniat, 12:*176-88, 1960.

411. LAGUAITE, J. K.: Techniques of therapy for laryngectomized patient. *South Speech J, 79:*86, 1957.

412. LALL, M., and EVISON, G.: Voice production following laryngopharyngo-esophagectomy with colon transplant. *J Laryng, 80:*1208-12, 1966.

413. LANDOIS und STRUERING, P.: Erzeugung einer Pseudo-Stimme bei einem Manne mit totaler Exstirpation des Kehlkopfes. *Arch Klin Chir, 38:* 143, 1889.

414. LARRU, E.: New orientations in the treatment of cancer of the larynx. *An Acad Nac Med (Madrid), 67:*3 1950.

415. LATKOWSKI, B., and OKON, J.: Niektóre dane statystyczne nowotworów zlosliwych krtani w polsce w latach 1956-1961. (Some statistical data on the malignant neoplasms of the larynx in Poland during the years 1956-1961. Summary.) *Otolaryng Pol, 19:*123, 1965.

416. LAUDER, E.: The role of the laryngectomee in post-laryngectomee voice instruction. *J Speech Hearing Dis, 30:*145-58, 1965.

417. LAVOIE, R.: Le cancer du larynx. *Laval Med, 18:*614-17, 1952.

418. LEDERER, F. L.: Audible speech following laryngectomie. *Arch Otolaryng (Chicago), 15:*947, 1932.

419. LEDERER, F. L.: *Diseases of the Ear, Nose and Throat.* Philadelphia, Davis, 1946.

420. LEGLER, U.: A new reliable way for rapid learning of an esophago-pharyngeal artificial voice for laryngectomized. *Arch Ohr Nas Kehl-kopfheilk, 162:*535-41, 1953.

421. LEHISTE, I., and PETERSON, G. E.: Linguistic considerations in the study of speech intelligibility. *J Acoust Soc Amer, 131:*250-86, 1959.

422. LE HUCHE, F.: Rééducation vocale du laryngectomise. (Vocal re-education after laryngectomy.) *France Med, 28:*275-78, 1965.

423. LEICHER, H.: Indikation und 5-Jahresheilungen bei radiochirurgischer Behandlung des Kehokopf- und Hypopharynxkarzinoms. (Indications and five year cures in radio-surgical treatment of laryngeal and hypopharyngeal carcinomas.) In Leroux-Robert, J. (Ed.): *Advances in Oto-Rhino-Laryngology.* Basel, S. Karger, 1961, pp. 220-74. Vol IX.

424. LEITNER, MARGARET ANN: A Study of the Effects of Intraphrase Rate and Pause Time on Information Gain and Speaker Image. Unpublished Ph.D. dissertation, University of Wisconsin, 1962.

425. LEJEUNE, F. E., SR.; STASSI, W., and LEJEUNE, F. E., JR.: Review of the available literature on the larynx for 1959. *Laryngoscope, 70:*1483-1522, 1960.

426. Le Quesne, L. P., and Ranger, D.: Pharyngolaryngectomy, with immeciate pharyngogastric anastomosis. *Brit J Surg, 53:*105-09, 1966.
427. Lerche, William: *The Esophagus and Pharynx in Action.* Springfield, Thomas, 1950.
428. Leroux, L., and Maspétiol: Partial horizontal laryngectomy in cancer of the base of the epiglottis. *Ann Otolaryng (Paris), 67:*663-72, 1950.
429. Leroux-Robert, J.: La chirugie seule et l'association chirurgieradiothérapie dans le traitement des épitheliomas du larynx et de l'hypopharnx. *Ann Otolaryng (Paris), 67:*217-66, 1950.
430. Leroux-Robert, J.: Laryngectomies partielles pour cancer du larynx; indications, techniques, résultats. *Ann. Otolaryng (Paris), 67:*5-15, 1950.
431. Leroux-Robert, J.: Indications et resultats apres 5 ans de la chirurgie conservatrice fonctionnelle des cancers du laryns et de l'hypopharynx. (Indications and results after 5 years of conservative functional surgery in cancer of the larynx and hypopharynx.) *Advances in Oto-Rhino-Laryngolosy.* Basel, S. Karger, 1961, Vol. 10, pp. 44-130.
432. Leroux-Robert, J.: Possibilitatile terapeutic si prognosticul cancerelor de laringe prin intermediul chirurgiei si al asocierilor radio-chirurgicale. In legatura cu o statistica personala de 1000 de cazuri operate in decurs de peste 5 ami. (Therapeutic possibilities in and the prognosis of cancers of the larynx treated by surgery or combined radiosurgery. With regard to a personal record of 1000 cases operated in more than five years.) *Otorhinolaryng Ruman, 10:*11-28, 1965.
433. Levin, N. M.: Laryngectomy. *Rehab Rec, 7:*13-14, 1966.
424. Leitner, Margaret Ann: A Study of the Effects of Intraphrase Rate and Voice Problems, Miami, Fla., June 1956.
435. Levin, N. M.: Recovering lost speech. *Rehab Rec, 6:*19-21, 1965.
436. Levin, N. M.: Rehabilitation after total laryngectomy. *Hear News, 32:* 9-13, 1964.
437. Levin, N. M.: Rehabilitation after total laryngectomy. In Anon., A Conference on Research Needs in the Rehabilitation of Persons with Disabilities Resulting from Cancer. New York, VRA and Inst. Phys. Med. Rehab., N.Y.U. Med Cent., 1966, pp. 55-71.
438. Levin, N. M.: Speech rehabilitation after total removal of larynx. *JAMA, 149:*1281-86, 1952.
439. Levin, N. M.: Teaching the laryngectomized patient to talk. *Arch Otolaryng (Chicago), 32:*299-314, 1940.
440. Levin, N. M.: Total laryngectomy and speech rehabilitation. *Eye Ear Nose Throat Monthly, 34:*585-92, 1955.
441. Levin, N. M. (Ed.) : *Voice and Speech Disorders: Medical Aspects.* Springfield, Thomas, 1962.
442. Lewis, D., and Tiffin, J.: A psychophysical study of individual differences in speaking ability. *Arch Sp, 1:*43-60, 1934.

443. LEWIS, F. O.: Laryngectomy with results in 17 cases. *Ann Otol, 33:*359-62, 1924.

444. LEYRO, DIAZ, J.: Laryngectomy and the artificial larynx. *Sem Méd (B. Aires), 31:*27, 1924.

445. Like teacher—like pupil. *IAL News, 6:*4, Feb. 1961.

446. LINDSAY, J. R.; MORGAN, R. H., and WEPMAN, J. M.: The cricopharyngeus muscle in esophageal speech. *Laryngoscope, 54:*55-65, 1944.

447. LINDSAY, JOHN K. (Ed.) : *1952 Yearbook of Eye, Ear, Nose and Throat.* Chicago, Year Bk, 1953.

448. LOEBELL, H., and BRAHM, K.: Gibt es beim Normalen einem Glottis-bzw. Sphinkterverschluss beim Heben von leichteren Gewichten (20 Kg.) und wie steht der Kehlkopftotalestirpierte den alltäglichen Balastungen gegenüber? *Folia Phoniat (Basel), 2:*67-68, 1950.

449. LUCHSINGER, R.: Beobachtungen u. Behandlung der Stimme nach chir.-röntgen. Therapie des Kehlkopfkrebses. *Schweiz Med Wschr, 50:* 561, 1939.

450. LUCHSINGER, R.: The mechanism of speech and voice training in the laryngectomy and exercise therapy. *Pract Otorhinolaryng (Basel), 14:* 304-23, 1952.

451. LUCHSINGER, R.: Phonetics and pathology. In Kaiser, L. (Ed.) : *Manual of Phonetics.* Amsterdam, North-Holland, 1957.

452. LUCHSINGER, R., and ARNOLD, G. E.: *Lehrbuch der Stimm-und Sprachheilkunde.* Vienna, Springer, 1949.

453. LUCHSINGER, R., and ARNOLD, G. E.: *Voice-Speech-Language. Clinical Communicology: Its Physiology and Pathology.* Belmont, Wadsworth, 1965.

454. LUEDERS, O. W.: Evaluation of post-laryngectomy rehabilitation program. *Arch Otolaryng (Chicago), 65:*572-74, 1957.

455. LUEDERS, O. W.: Use of the electrolarynx in speech rehabilitation. *Arch Otolaryng (Chicago), 63:*133-34, 1956.

456. LYNCH, J.: *Choose to Speak.* Austin Texas Division, American Cancer Soc., 1962, p. 16.

457. MAAS, H.: Exstirpation des Kehlkopfes, Heilung. *Arch Klin Chir, 20:* 535-39, 1876.

458. MACONIE, A. C.: Diagnosis and modern treatment of malignant diseases of the larynx. *Med Press, 225:*77-81, 1951.

459. MACKENSIE, M.: *Diseases of the Pharynx, Larynx, and Trachea.* New York, William Wood, 1880.

460. MACKENTY, J. E.: Cancer of larynx. *Arch Otolaryng (Chicago), 3:*205-32, 1926; cont. *3:*305-37, 1926.

461. MACKENTY, J. E.: Laryngectomy with good speaking voice. *Laryngoscope, 30:*112, 1920.

462. MACKENTY, J. E.: Laryngectomy in one stage. *Surg Gynec Obstet, 42:* 644-51, 1926.

463. MacKenty, J. E.: Operation after total laryngectomy for cure of intrinsic cancer of the larynx. *Ann Otol, 31:*1101-17, 1922.

464. MacKenty, J. E.: Technique and after treatment of hemilaryngectomy and laryngectomy. *JAMA, 69:*863-69, 1917.

465. Malbeck, E., and Schlosshauer, B.: Phoniatrische nachuntersuchungen chordektomierter patienten. (Phoniatric examinations of cordectomized patients.) *HNO, 8:*201-05, 1960.

466. Mantinez Moncunill, A.: Posibilidades de la cirugiá parcial en el cancer de la laringe. (Possibilities of partial surgery of cancer of the larynx.) *Rev Otorhinolaryng, 23:*21-26, 1963.

467. Marco, J.; Morera, H., and Gimenez, J. A.: Olfaction in laryngectomy. *Rev Esp Otoneuooftal, 13:*76, 380-94, 1954.

468. Marland, P. M.: A direct method of teaching voice after total laryngectomy. *Speech, 13:*4-13, 1949.

469. Marley, F.: Cancer victims speak again. *Science News Letter,* July 23, 1960.

470. Marley, F.: They speak again in triumph. *New York World-Telegram,* (Feature Magazine Section), June 25, 1960.

471. Marschik, H., and Fröschels, E.: Fall von Total-exstirpation des Kehlkopfes. Pharynxstimme u. Oesophagusatmung. *Mschr Ohrenheilk, 63:*581, 1929.

472. Martin, H.: Esophageal speech. *Ann Otol, 59:*687-89, 1950.

473. Martin, H.: Incidence of total laryngectomy. *Ann Otol, 59:*359, 1950.

474. Martin, H.: Rehabilitation of the laryngectomee. *CA, 1:*147-52, 1951.

475. Martin, H.: Selection of treatment in cancer of the larynx. *Ann Otol, 50:*723-34, 1941.

476. Martin, H.: Speech rehabilitation following laryngectomy; general consideration. *Talk, 36:*4-6, 1955.

477. Martin, H.: Rehabilitation of the laryngectomee. *Cancer, 16:*823-41, 1963.

478. Marx: Patient mit pharynx-und Larystimme. *Med Klin, 22:*1127, 1926.

479. Mason, M.: The rehabilitation of patients following surgical removal of the larynx. *J Laryng, 64:*759-70, 1950.

480. Matzker, J., and Thelen, P. O.: Über die Funktion der Bauchpresse bie fehlendem Glottisschluss. *Z Laryng Rhinol, 34:*819-25, 1955.

481. McCall, J. W.: Preliminary voice training for laryngectomy. *Arch Otolaryng (Chicago), 38:*10-16, 1943.

482. McCall, J. W.: Preoperative training for development of the esophageal voice in laryngectomized patients. *Ann Otol, 52:*364-76, 1943.

483. McCall, J. W.; Dixon, L., and Hoerr, N.: The mucous membranes after laryngectomy. *Ann Otol, 58:*535, 1949.

484. McCall, J. W., and Fisher, R.: Carcinoma of the larynx. A report of 194 cases with 149 laryngectomies. *Arch Otolaryng (Chicago), 62:*475, 1952.

485. McCALL, J. W., and STOVER, W. C.: Laryngectomy for laryngeal cancer; a review of 45 cases. *Laryngoscope, 54:*659-76, 1944.

486. McCALL, J. W., and WHITAKER, C. W.: The use of prostheses in the larynx and trachea. A preliminary report. *Ann Otol, 71:*397-403, 1962.

487. McCASKEY, C. H.: Voice apparatus in laryngectomized patients. *Trans Indiana Acad Ophth Otolaryng, 23:*44-47, 1940.

488. McCLEAR, JOHN: A new voice for the laryngectomized. *RN, 22:*40-43, 1959.

489. McCLEAR, J. E.: *Esophageal Voice Production.* An instruction manual. New York, National Hospital for Speech Disorders, 61 Irving Place, 1960.

490. McCROSKEY, R. L., and MULLIGAN, M.: The relative intelligibility of esophageal speech and artificial-larynx speech. *J Speech Hearing Dis, 28:*37-41, 1963.

491. McKESSON, E. I. A.: A mechanical larynx. *JAMA, 88:*645, 1927.

492. McKINLEY, S.: Correlates of Stress Patterns in Esophageal Speech. Unpublished master's thesis, Vanderbilt University, 1960.

493. MEAD, J.; McILROY, M. B.; SELVERSTONE, N. J., and KREITE, B. C.: Measurement of intraesophageal pressure. *J Appl Physiol, 7:*491-95, 1955.

494. METFESSEL, M.: Techniques for the objective study of vocal art. *Psychol Monogr, 36:*1-40, 1927.

495. MEYER, R.: Patient mit total exstirpierten Larynx und kuenslichem Kehlkopf. *Berl Klin Wschr, 47:*35, 1910.

496. MICHELI-PELLEGRINI, V.: On the so-called pseudo-glottis in laryngectomized persons. *J Laryng, 71:*405, 1957.

497. MICHELI-PELLEGRINI, V., and FINISTORCHI, O.: Importanza della "labiovibrazione" nella reeducazione dei laringectomizzati. (Importance of "labiovibration" in the reeduction of laryngectomees.) *Bol Mal Orecch, 82:*28-35, 1964.

498. MICHELI-PELLEGRINI, V., and RAGAGLINI, G.: Richerche sulla fonazione dei laringectomizzati. (Research on phonation of laryngectomized patients.) *Boll Mal Orecch, 69:*506-09, 1951.

499. MIKELL, J. S.; NEFFERSON, A. H., and DALY, C. A.: Neurofibroma of the larynx in a 5 yr. old child; laryngectomy, rehabilitation. *Ariz Med, 11:*167-68, 1954.

500. MIKICHI: Recherches morphologiques de l'influence de la pharyngectomie et de la laryngectomie sur la muqueuse nasale. *Zibi Intoka Rinzyo, 49:*890, 1956.

501. MILLER, ALDEN H.: First experiences with the Asai technique for vocal rehabilitation after total laryngectomy. *Ann Otol, 76:*829-33, 1967.

502. MILLER, DANIEL: Psychological consideration in the management of cancer. *Ann Otol, 69:*236-44, 1960.

503. MILLER, M. H.: The responsibility of the speech therapist to the laryngectomized patient. *Arch Otolaryng (Chicago), 70:*211-16, 1959.

504. MILLER, W.: Esophageal speech solves a problem. *J Rehab, 17*:7-9, 1951.
505. MINIFIE, F. D.: An Analysis of the Durational Aspects of Connected Speech Samples by Means of an Electronic Speech Duration Analyzer. Unpublished Ph.D. dissertation, State University of Iowa, 1963.
506. MIODONSKI, J.: Hemilaryngektomia rozszerzoma. (Extended hemilaryngectory.) *Otolaryng Pol, 17*:9-14, 1963.
507. MIRAGLIA DEL GIUDICE, E.; AMORELLI, A., and PERRELLA, F.; Rilievi audiometrici in soggetti laringectomizzati. (Audiometric findings in laryngectomees.) *Arch Ital Laring, 69*:277-92.
508. MÖCKEL, G., and SCHLOSSHAUER, B.: Speech in the absence of a larynx; roentgencinematographic analysis of the pseudo-speech of laryngectomized patients. *Deutsch Med Wschr, 80*:1244-46, 1955.
509. MONTEIRO, L.: The patient had difficulty communicating. *Amer J Nurs, 62*:78-81, 1962.
510. MONTREUIL, F.: Cancer of the larynx. *Canad Med Ass J, 82*:1216-19, 1960.
511. MONTREUIL, F.: Cancer of the larynx: early diagnosis and rehabilitation. *Un Med Canada, 83*:649-55, 1954.
512. MOOLENAAR-BIJL, A. J.: Connection between consonant articulation and the intake of air in oesophageal speech. *Folia Phoniat (Basel), 5*:212-15, 1953.
513. MOOLENAAR-BIJL, A. J.: De spraak na larynxextirpatie. *Nederl T Geneesk, 97*:2379, 1953.
514. MOOLENAAR-BIJL, A. J.: Larynxlozen spreken weer. *T V Log en Phon,* 1950.
515. MOOLENAAR-BIJL, A. J.: Some data on speech without larynx. *Folia Phonit (Basel), 3:1*:20-24, 1951.
516. MOOLENAAR-BIJL, A. J.: Sprenken zonder larynx. *Nederl T Geneesk, 91*: 118, 1947.
517. MOOLENAAR-BIJL, A. J.: The importance of certain consonants in oesophageal voice after laryngectomy. *Ann Otol, 62*:979, 1953.
518. MOORE, G. P.: Voice disorders associated with organic abnormalities. In Travis, L. E. (Ed.): *Handbook of Speech Pathology.* New York, Appleton, 1957.
519. MOORE, G. P.; WHITE, F. D., and VON LEDEN, H.: Ultra high speed photography in laryngeal physiology. *J Speech Hearing Dis, 27*:165-71, 1962.
520. MORRISON, W. W.: Physical rehabilitation of the laryngectomized patient. *Arch Otolaryng (Chicago), 34*:1101-12, 1941.
521. MORRISON, W. W.: The production of voice and speech after total laryngectomy. *Arch Otolaryng (Chicago), 14*:413-23, 1931.
522. MORRISON, W. W., and FINEMAN, S.: The production of the pseudovoice after total laryngectomy. *Trans Amer Acad Ophth Otolaryng, 41*: 631-34, 1936.

523. Mosciaro, O., and Sassi, P.: La deglutizione nelle laringectomie orizzontali. (Swallowing following horizontal laryngectomy.) *Otorhinolaring Ital, 35:*123-33, 1966.

524. Moses, P. J.: Rehabilitation of the post-laryngectomized patient; the vocal therapist and contribution to the rehabilitation program. *Ann Otol, 67:*538-43, 1958.

525. Mosher, H. P.: X-ray study of movements of the tongue, epiglottis, and hyoid bone in swallowing. *Laryngoscope, 37:*235-62, 1927.

526. Motta, G.; Profazio, A., and Acciarri, T.: Osservasioni roentgencinematografiche sulla fonazione nei laringectomizzati. (Roentgenocinematographic observations on the phonation of laryngectomized subjects.) *Otorinolaring Ital, 28:*261-86, 1959.

527. Moulonguet, A., et Garde, E. J.: La rééducation de la voix chez les laryngectomisés. *Ann Otolaryng (Paris), 61:*70, 1944.

528. Mounier-Kuhn, P.; Gaillard, J., and Charachon, R.: Indications de la chirurgie laryngee horizontale sus glottique. (Indications for supraglottal horizontal laryngeal surgery.) *J Franc Otorinolaring, 13:*783-96, 1964.

529. Mounier-Kuhn, P.; Gaillard, J.; Morgon, A., and Fontvie-Ille, J.: Hemilaryngectomie pour angiome géant du larynx. (Hemilaryngectomy for giant angioma of the larynx.) *J Franc Otorinolaring, 10:*1030-35, 1961.

530. Murphy, G. E.; Bisno, A. L., and Ogura, J. H.: Determinants of rehabilitation following laryngectomy. *Laryngoscope, 74:*1535-49, 1964.

531. Nadell, A.: Electronics helps the mute to speak. *Radio Electronics,* June 1959.

532. Nadoleczny, M.: Was muss der Hals-Nasen-Ohrenarzt von Sprach-und Stimmheilkunde wissen? *Z Hals Ohrenheilk, 44:*1-74, 1938.

533. Nahum, A. M., and Golden, J. S.: Psychological problems of laryngectomy. *JAMA, 186:*1136-38, 1963.

534. Negus, V. E.: Affectations of the cricopharyngeal fold. *Laryngoscope, 48:*847-58, 1938.

535. Negus, V. E.: *The Comparative Anatomy and Physiology of the Larynx.* London, W. Heinemann, 1949.

536. Negus, V. E.: Restoration of speech after removal of the larynx. *Cesk Otolaryng, 5:*5-12, 1956.

537. Negus, V. E.: The second stage of swallowing. *Acta Otolaryng (Stockholm),* (suppl.), pp. 76-81, 1948-49.

538. Nelson, C. R.: You can speak again. *Post Laryngectomy Speech.* New York, Funk, 1949.

539. Nessel, E.: Künstliche Kehlköpfe. (Artificial larynx.) *HNO, 11:*249-53, 1963.

540. Neuberger, F.: On psychology and sociology of the laryngectomee. *Mschr Ohrenheilk, 85:*198-218, 1951.

541. New, G. B.: Summary of cancer of the larynx. *Laryngoscope, 61*:523-29, 1951.

542. Nichols, A. C.: Power spectra of the pre- and postoperative speech of a laryngectomee. *Asha, 1*:105, 1959. Abstract of a paper presented to the American Speech and Hearing Association, New York, November, 1959.

543. Nightingale, E. J.; Svigals, C.; Mersheimer, N. L., and Boyd, L. J.: Some important clinical aspects of esophageal carcinoma; an analysis of 413 cases. *Amer J Dig Dis, 21*:341-53, 1954.

544. Norris, C. M.: Rehabilitation of the post-laryngectomized patient. 1. Types of clinical cases and their resultant esophageal, pharyngeal, and neck deformities. *Ann Otol, 67*:528-37, 1958.

545. Norris, C. M.: Technique of extended fronto-lateral partial laryngectomies. *Laryngoscope, 68*:1240-50, 1958.

546. Novotny, O.: Late results of larynx extirpation after radiotherapy. *Mschr Ohrenheilk, 89*:126-30, 1955.

547. Nursing care after laryngectomy. *Cancer Bull (Houston), 11*:28-29, 1959.

548. Nussdorfer, R.: Late results in laryngectomy, social problems of laryngectomized persons. *Otorinolaring Ital, 12*:366-75, 1942.

549. Nylen, C. O., and Drettner, B.: Esophageal speech and ventriloquism. *Pract Otorhinolaryng (Basel), 19*:570-75, 1957.

550. Obreja, S., and Pacuraru, I.: Limitele indicatiei chirurgicale in cancerul de laringe. (Limits of surgical indications in cancer of the larynx. *Otornolaryng Ruman, 3*:257-62, 1962.

551. Ogura, J. H.: Laryngectomy and radical neck dissection for cancer of the larynx. *Trans Amer Acad Ophth Otolaryng, 56*:786, 1951.

552. Ogura, J. H.: Supraglottic subtotal laryngectomy and neck dissection. *Laryngoscope, 68*:983-1003, 1958.

553. Ogura, J. H.; Shumrick, D. A., and Lapidot, A.: Some observations on experimental laryngeal substitution in laryngectomized dogs. *Ann Otol, 71*:532-50, 1962.

554. Ogura, Joseph, and Bello, J.: Laryngectomy and radical neck dissection for carcinoma of the larynx. *Laryngoscope, 62*:1-52, 1952.

555. Ombrédanne, M.: *Traitement du cancer edolaryngé.* Paris, Masson et Cié, 1930.

556. Onodi, A.: Ergebnisse der Abteilung fuer Hoer-Sprach-Stimmstoerungen und Tracheotomierte. *Mschr Ohrenheilk, 52*:85, 1918.

557. Oppenheim, H.: Lower airway obstruction after laryngectomy. *Ear Eye Nose Throat Monthly, 43*:66-68, 1964.

558. Oreskovic, M.: La chirurgie conservatrice du larynx et la phonation. (Conservative surgical intervention of the larynx and phonation.) *Folia Phoniat, 14*:280-87, 1962.

559. Oreskovic, M.: La voix après cordectomie. (The voice after cordectomy.) *Rev Laryng (Bordeaux), 80*:301-17, 1959.

560. ORLANDI, G.: La laringectomia parziale orizzontale. (Partial horizontal laryngectomy.) *Arch Ital Otol, 73:*940-61, 1962.

561. ORMEROD, F. C.: The indications for and the five year results of surgery of cancer of the hypopharynx. In Leroux-Robert, J. (Ed.) : *Advances in Oto-Rhino-Laryngology.* Basel, S. Karger, 1961, vol. 10, pp. 193-219.

562. ORMEROD, F. C.: Partial pharyngolaryngectomy with primary sleeve-graft reconstruction. *J Laryng, 71:*175-201, 1957.

563. ORTON, H. B.: Cancer of the larynx. *Arch Otolaryng (Chicago), 28:* 153, 1938.

564. ORTON, H. B.: A review of the available literature on the larynx and laryngeal surgery. *Laryngoscope, 62:*181-205, 1948.

565. ORTON, H. B.: Review of diseases of the larynx. *Laryngoscope, 50:*158-63, 1940.

566. ORTON, H. B.: Treatment of extensive carcinoma of the larynx. *Laryngoscope, 59:*496-510, 1951.

567. OSBORNE, A.: My experience of laryngectomies and esophageal speech. *J Logopedics, 1:*20-23, 1950.

568. OTTOSSON, B. G.: Myoblastoma of the larynx. *Acta Otolaryng (Stockholm), 58:*87-93, 1964.

569. PADDOCK, M. A.: Scaled Samples of Defective Voice for Listener Training. Unpublished M.A. thesis, San Diego State College, 1967.

570. PANCOAST, H. K.; PENDERGRASS, E. P., and SCHAEFFER, J. P.: *Head and Neck in Roentgen Diagnosis.* Springfield, Thomas, 1940, p. 864.

571. PANCONCELLI-CALZIA, G.: *Geschichtszahlen der Phonetik.* Hamburg, Hansischer Gildenverlag, 1941.

572. PANCONCELLI-CALZIA, G.: *Quellanatlas zur Geschichte der Phonetik.* Hamburg, Hansischer Gildenverlag, 1940.

573. PANCONCELLI-CALZIA, G.: The value of the Lombard reaction in laryngectomized patients. *Acta Otolaryng (Stockholm), 49:*162-64, 1958.

574. PANTIUKHIN, V. P.: Stroboskopia u bol'nykh posle laringektomii. (Stroboscopy in patients following laryngectomy.) *Vestn Otorinolaring, 23:*69-73, 1961.

575. PELLEGRINI, V. M.: Causes that might prevent the phonetic re-education of laryngectomized. *Boll Mal Orecch, 75:*399-408, 1957.

575. PELLEGRINI, V. M.: On the so-called pseudoglottis in laryngectomized persons. *J Laryng, 71:*405-10, 1957.

577. PELLEGRINI, V. M.: Phonetic possibilities of laryngectomized patient. *Boll Mal Orecch, 77:*19-24, 1959.

578. PELLEGRINI, V. M., and RAGAGLINI, G.: Studies on phonation in laryngectomized. *Boll Mal Orecch, 69:*493-545, 1951.

579. PELLEGRINI, V. M., and RAGAGLINI, G.: Further data on phonation of laryngectomees. *Boll Mal Orecch, 72:*365-73, 1954.

580. PERELLÓ, J.: La educacion foniátrica de los laryngectomizdos. *Med Clin (Barcelona), 17:*251-53, 1951.

581. PERELLÓ, J.: Prognosis in voice building. *Acta Otorinolaring Iber Amer,* 8:248-54, 1957.

582. PERELLÓ, J.: El Pronóstico en la Erigmofonía. Proceedings Tenth Inter. Speech Voice Conf. Barcelona, 1957.

583. PERELLÓ, J.: Les resultats de l'erygmophonie. *J France Otorinolaring, 10:* 1, 1961.

584. PERELLÓ, J.: Les techniques chirurgicales dans la laryngectomie et le resultat erygmophonique. (Surgical techniques in laryngectomy and the resulting esophageal voice.) *J Franc Otorinolaring, 12:67-69,* 1963.

585. PERELLÓ, J.: La voix du laryngectomisé. En *La Voix.* Paris, Maloine, 1953.

586. PERRON, R.; MAZAURIC, F., and MANIPOUD, J.: Chondro-sarcome du larynx. (Chondro-sarcoma of the larynx.) *J Franc Otorinolaring, 16:* 257-59, 1967.

587. PERRY, P. S.: An Investigation of the Lowest Frequency in Normal and Esophageal Vowel Phonation. Unpublished Ph.D. dissertation, University of Michigan, 1963.

588. PESAVENTO, G.: La ricostruzione dell'esofago cervicale dopo faringo-laringectomia totale. (The reconstruction of the cervical esophagus after total pharyngolaryngectomy.) *Minerva Otorinolaring, 11:200-* 04, 1961.

589. PETERSEN, A.: Über das Postoperative Schicksal der Kahlkopfextirpierten. Dissertation, Kiel, 1952.

590. PETERSON, G. E.: Breath stream dynamics and articulation. In Kaiser, L. (Ed.): *Manual of Phonetics.* Amsterdam, North-Holland, 1957.

591. PICHLER, H. J.: Über ein Neuarti ges Automatisch Gesteuertes Elektronisches Sperechgerät für Laryngektomierte. *Acta Otolaryng (Stockholm),* 53:374-80, 1961.

592. PIERANGELI, C.: L'importanza del rinfornimento inspiratorio dell esofago nella voce dei laringectomizzati. *Arch Ital Mal Trach, 10:16,* 1942.

593. PIQUET, J.: Reeducation and social rehabilitation of laryngectomized. *Bull Acad Nat Méd (Paris), 138:232-34,* 1954.

594. PODVINEC, J.: Entstchung der Sprache bei Tracheotomierten und Laryngektomierten. *Otolaryng Slav, 4:*1932.

595. POMMEZ, J. M. E.: Voix Oesophagienne Après Laryngectomie Totale. Thèse Bordeaux, 1952-53.

596. POPPERT: Zur Frage der totalen Kehlkopfexstirpation. *Deutsch Med Wschr, 19:*833, 1893.

597. PORTMANN, M., and POMMEZ, J.: Esophageal voice. *J Méd (Bordeaux),* 129:495-99, 1952.

598. PRECETHEL, A.: Reconstitution fonctionelle de la pseudoglotte oesophagienne dans la laryngectomie. *Acta Otorhinolaryng (Belg.), 6:* 550-58, 1958.

599. PRECETHEL, A.: La Stroboscopie dans le diagnostic precoce du cancer de la corde vocale. (Stroboscopy for early diagnosis of cancer of the vocal cord.) *Arch Ital Otol, 72*:299-310, 1961.

600. PRESSMAN, J. J.: The action of the larynx. *Proc Roy Soc Med J Laryng Otol, 53*:672, 1938.

601. PRESSMAN, J. J.: Cancer of the larynx — laryngoplasto to avoid laryngectomy. *Arch Otolaryng (Chicago), 59*:395-412, 1954.

602. PRESSMAN, J. J.: Physiology of the larynx. A resume and discussion of the literature for 1938. *Laryngoscope, 49*:1-21, 1939.

603. PRESSMAN, J. J., and SIMON, M. B.: Tracheal stretching and metaplasia of the tracheal rings from cartilage to bone following the use of aortic homografts. *Amer Surg, 25*:850-56, 1959.

604. Proceedings, First Institute on Voice Pathology and First International Meeting of Laryngectomized Persons, Cleveland Hearing and Speech Center, August 1-2, 1952, Cleveland, Ohio.

605. PRUSZEWICZ, A., and OBREBOWSKI, A.: Zachowanie sie powonienia i smaku u chorych po calkowitym wyluszczeniu krtani. (The behavior of the sense of smell and taste in patients after radical laryngectomy.) *Atolaryng Pol, 20*:425-29, 1966.

606. PTACEK, P. H., and SANDER, E. K.: Maximum duration of phonation. *J Speech Res, 28*:171-82, 1963.

607. PUTNEY, F. J.: Rehabilitation of the post-laryngectomized patient; specific discussion of failures; advanced and difficult technical problems. *Ann Otol, 67*:544-49, 1958.

608. RAGAGLINI, C.; TERAMO, M., and MICHELI-PELLEGRINI, V.: Further cineradiograph research in the study of the phonation of laryngectomized patient. Extract from *Nunt Radiol, 22*:156-63, 1956.

609. RAGAGLINI, C.; TERAMO, M., and MICHELI-PELLEGRINI, V.: La rontgencinematografia nello studio della voce dei laringectomizzati. (Cineradiographic study of the voice in laryngectomized patients.) *Nunt Radiol, 21*:127-31, 1955.

610. RAGAGLINI, C.; TERAMO, M., and MICHELI-PELLEGRINI, V.: La voce a-laringea. (Alaryngeal voice.) *Radiol Med (Torino), 11* (n. 11), Nov. 1955.

611. RAMSEY, G. H.; WATSON, J. S.; GRAMIAK, R., and WEINBERG, S. A.: Cineflurographic analysis of the mechanism of swallowing. *Radiology, 64*:498-518, 1955.

612. RASMUSSEN, H., and SØRENSEN, K.: Partial laryngectomy in the treatment of cancer of the larynx. *Acta Otolaryng (Stockholm), 58*:68-72, 1964.

613. REED, G. F.: The long-term follow-up care of laryngectomized patients. *JAMA, 174*:980-85, 1961.

614. REED, G. F., and SNOW, J. B., JR.: Reappraisal of seventy-five cases of radical neck dissection for carcinoma of the larynx. *Ann Otol, 69*:271-79, 1960.

615. REICHARD, W.: The rehabilitation of the laryngectomized patient. *Bol Asoc Mèd P Rico, 46:*162-67, 1954.

616. Report of the American Cancer Society and International Association of Laryngectomees, October 13, 1955.

617. 'Reverse hearing aid' aids laryngectomees. *Scope Weekly, 3:*5 (Dec 24) 1958.

618. REYHER, C.: Die Laryngostrictur und ihre Heilung durch den kuenstlichen Kehlkopf. *Arch Klin Chir, 19:*334, 1876.

619. REYNAUD, M.: Observation sur une fistule aerienne, avec occlusion complete de la partie inferieure du larynx, pour servir a l'histoire de la phonation. *Gaz Med Paris, 9* (ser. II) :583, 1841.

620. RICKENBERG, H. E.: Laryngectomized speech. *Arch Otolaryng (Chicago), 58:*421-24, 1953.

621. RIESZ, R. R.: Description and demonstration of an artificial larynx. *J Acoust Soc Amer, 1:*273, 1930.

622. ROBE, E. Y.; MOORE, P.; ANDREWS, A. H., JR., and HOLINGER, P. H.: A study of the role of certain factors in the development of speech after laryngectomy. 1. Type of operation. *Laryngoscope, 66:*173-86, 1956; 2. Site of pseudoglottis. *Laryngoscope, 66:*382-401, 1956; 3. Coordination of speech with respiration. *Laryngoscope, 66:*481-99, 1956.

623. ROBERTS, R. I.: A cineradiographic investigation of pharyngeal deglutition. *Brit J Radiol, 30:*449-60, 1957.

624. ROGERS, W. P., JR.; REYNOLDS, C., and YATSUHASHI, M.: Cancer of the larynx. *New Eng J Med, 274:*596-99, 1966.

625. ROLLIN, W. J.: A Comparative Study of Vowel Formants of Esophageal and Normal-speaking Adults. Unpublished Ph.D. dissertation, Wayne State University, 1962.

626. ROMONEK, P. L.: Artificial and pseudo-voice following complete laryngectomy. *Nebraska Med J, 17:*238-43, 1932.

627. ROMENEK, P. L.: Reeducation of the voice following a complete laryngectomy for carcinoma of the larynx. *Trans Amer Laryng Rhino Otol Soc, 37:*514-17, 1931.

628. ROSEDALE, R.: Laryngectomy. *Ohio Speech and Hearing Therapist, 1:*1, 1950.

629. ROUSSELOT, P.: La parole avec un larynx artificiel. *La Parole, 12:*1902.

630. ROVNICK, S., and SOKOLOW,, E.: A case work experience with patients following loss of larynx. *Rehab Lit, 26:*135-39, 1965.

631. RUBALTELLI: Assistenza medica e humana al laringectomizzato. *Ann Laring, 55:*405, 1957.

632. RUBIN, H.: High-speed cinematography of the pathologic larynx. Cedars of Lebanon Hospital, Los Angeles, California, 1959.

633. RUBIN, H.: Ultra High Speed Motion Pictures of the Esophagus. ASHA Convention Report, 1960.

634. SAKU, Y.: Statistical observation and frequency analysis studies of

artificial larynges. (Japanese text.) *Otol Fukuoka (Fukuoka), 5:*101-16, 1959.

635. SARTORIO, C.; BOCCA, E., and BOZZANI, V.: Controllo radiologico del luego di formazione della Pseudoglottide in Laryngectomizati rieducatti (Nota preliminare). *Boll Soc Ital Fon Sperimentale,* Nov. 1950.

636. SAUNDERS, J. B. DEC.; DAVIS, C., and MILLER, E. R.: The mechanism of deglutition (second stage) as revealed by cineradiography. *Ann Otol, 60:*897-916, 1951.

637. SCHAER, A.: Bibliographisches Referat über Stimme und Sprache der Laryngektomierten (1898-1923). Manuskr. Phonet. Lab. Univ. Hamburg. Registrierung oesophagealer Phonationsbewegungen, 1927.

638. SCHALL, L. A.: Cancer of the larynx: In *Cancer — A Manual for Practitioners,* 3rd ed. Boston, Amer Cancer Society (Mass. Division) Inc. 1956, pp. 166-69.

639. SCHALL, L. A.: Psychology of laryngectomized patients. *Arch Otolaryng (Chicago), 28:*581-84, 1938.

640. SCHILLING, R., and BINDER, H.: Experimental-phonetische Untersuchunger über die Stimme ohne Kehlkopf. *Arch Ohr Nas Kohlkopfheilk, 115:*235, 1926.

641. SCHILLING, R., and BINDER, H.: Über die Pharynx-und Oesophagusstimme. *Zbl Hals Nas Ohrenheilk, 9:*893, 1927.

642. SCHLORHAUFER, W.: Contribution to the esophageal speech. *Z Laryng Rhinol Otol, 34:*2:91-94, 1955.

643. SCHLOSSHAUER, B., and MOCKEL, G.: Answertung der Rontgentonfilm von Speiserohrensprechern. (Interpretation of roentgen sound films of esophageal speakers). *Folia Phoniat, 10:*154-66, 1958.

644. SCHLOSSHAUER, B.: Rontgenkinematografische Darstellung der Pseudosprache nach Laryngektomie. *Arch Ohr Nas Kehlkopfheilk, 165:* 581, 638, 1954.

645. SCHMID, H.: Zur Statistik des totalexstirpation des Kehlkopfes im funktionellem sinne: laute, verständliche Sprache. *Arch Klin Chir, 38:* 132-42, 1888-9.

646. SCHMUGGE, R. E.: Laryngectomies and tracheotomies. Training Bulletin, Training Division, Fire Department, St. Paul, Minn.

647. SCHÖNHÄRL, E.: Vergleichende sonagraphische Vokalanalysen unter Verwendung des "kunstlichen elektronishchen Kehlkopfes." (Comparative sonographic vocal analysis using the artificial electronic larynx.) *Z Laryng Rhinol Otol, 41:*845-47, 1962.

648. SCHOTT, L. O.; An electrical vocal system. *Bell Lab Record, 28:*549, 1950.

649. SCHULTHESS, G. VON: Temperature measurements in the respiratory tract of laryngectomized patients. *Acta Otolaryng (Stockholm), 57:* 325-31, 1964.

650. SCHWAB, W.: Cineradiographic research on post-laryngectomy speech. *Acta Otorinolaring Iber Amer, 8:*270-73, 1957.

651. SCHWAB, W.: Morphological and functional changes at the respiratory tract after laryngectomy. *Arch Ohr Nas Kehlkopfheilk, 166*:444-75, 1955.

652. SCHWAB, W.: Radiography and cinematography of the upper esophagus after laryngectomy. *Arch Ohr Nas Kehlkopfheilk, 169*:301-03, 1956.

653. SCHWAB, W.: Roentgen cinematographic studies on substitute speech after laryngectomy. *Krebsarzt, 13*:236-38, 1958.

654. SCHWAB, W.: The x-ray appearance of the hypopharynx in laryngectomized subject. *Arch Ohr Nas Kehlkopfheilk, 167*:521-24, 1955.

655. SCHWARTZ, A. W., and DEVINE, K. D.: Some historical notes about the first laryngectomies. *Laryngoscope, 69*:194-201, 1959.

656. SCRIPTURE, E. W.: Speech without a larynx. *JAMA, 60*:1601, 1913 .

657. SCRIPTURE, E. W.: Speech without using the larynx. *J Physiol, 50*:397-403, 1915-1916.

658. SCUDERI, R.: Variations of the temperature of the air on the trachea of laryngectomized. *Boll Soc Ital Biol Sper, 27*:818-20, 1951.

659. SCURI, D.: Importance of conservation of epiglottis in laryngectomy for eventual reeducation of speech. *Arch Ital Otol, 41*:18-34, 1930.

660. SCURI, D.: Meccanismo fonetico nei laringectomizzati. *Arch Ital Otol, 42*:318-37, 1931.

661. SCURI, D.: Reeducation after laryngectomy. *Arch Ital Otol, 41*:577-84, 1930.

662. SCURI, D.: L'assistenza foniatrica dei laringectomizzati. (Phoniatric therapy of the laryngectomized.) *Udito Voce Parola, 4*:327-33, 1961.

663. SEDLÁCEK, K.: Predni a laterálni rekonstrukcni laryngektomie se staženim epiglottis. (Reconstructive anterior and lateral laryngectomy using the epiglottis as a pedunculated graft.) *Cesk Otolaryng, 14*:328-34, 1965.

664. SEEMAN, M.: Movements of esophagus in phonation. *Cas lek Cesk, 63*:771-76, 984-94, 1011-21, 1924.

665. SEEMAN, M.: Registrierung oesophagealer phonationsbewegungen. *Vox, 9*:1927; Obstrated i n*JAMA, 83*:484, 1924.

666. SEEMAN, M.: Pathology of the esophageal voice. *Folia Phoniat (Basel), 10*:44-50, 1958.*

667. SEEMAN, M.: Phoniatrische Bemerkungen zu Laryngektomie. *Arch Klin Chir, 140*:285-98, 1926.

668. SEEMAN, M.: Speech and voice without larynx. *Cas lek Cesk, 61*:369-72, 1922.

669. SEEMAN, M.: Speech rehabilitation following laryngectomy. *Cas lek Cesk, 90*:1359-64, 1951.

670. SEGRE, R., Y ARDISSONE: Protesis mecanica para la fonacion de los laringectomizados. *Acta Otorinolaring Iber Amer, 4*:169, 1950.

671. SEIFFERT, A.: Bildung einer Pseudoglottis bei einew Laryngektomierten. *Z Laryng usw, 19*:358, 1930.

672. SEILER, C.: A case of laryngeal stenosis with audible articulation. *Philad Med Times, 18:*199, 1888.

673. SERCER, A.: The voice after plastic reconstruction of the lumen of the larynx. *Rev Laryng (Bordeaux), 80:*642-65, 1959.

674. SERGIO URRUTIA, C.: Cirugia del cáncer de la laringe. (Surgery of laryngeal cancer.) *Rev Otorrinolaring (Santiago), 22:*15-22, 1962.

675. SERGIO URRUTIA, C., and SALAMANCA, A.: Reconstruccion plastica faringoesofagica en cancer laringofaringeo extenso. (Plastic-pharynx reconstruction in extensive larynx-pharynx cancer.) *Rev Otorrinolaring (Santiago), 24:*60-62, 1964.

676. SERRA, M.: Osservazioni su 1,977 laringectomizzati sottoposti a rieducazione ortofonica. (Obeservations on 1,977 laryngectomees who underwent speech therapy.) *Arch Ital Laring, 70:*401-13, 1962.

677. SHAMES, G. H.; FONT, J., and MATTHEWS, J.: Factors related to speech proficiency of the laryngectomized. *J Speech Hearing Dis, 28:*273-87, 1963.

678. SHAMES, G. H.; MATTHEWS, J., and FONT, J.: A Study of Factors Related to the Learning of Post-laryngectomized Speech. Vocational Rehabilitation Administration, Department of Health, Education and Welfare, Project Number 465, 1962.

679. SHANKS, J. C.: Advantages in the use of esophageal speech by a laryngectomee. *Laryngoscope, 77:*239-43, 1967.

680. SHEARD, C.: Production of speech after laryngectomy. *Surg Clin N Amer, 12:*959-65, 1932.

681. SHELTON, R. L., JR.; BROOKS, ALTA; DIEDRICH, W. M.; YOUNGSTROM, K., and BROOKS, R. S.: Filming speed in cineflurographic speech study. *J Speech Hearing Dis, 6:*19-26, 1963.

682. SHELTON, R. L., JR.; DIEDRICH, W. M., and YOUNGSTROM, K.: The evaluation of speech mechanisms. *J Kansas Med Soc, 62:*396-99, 1961.

683. SHIBATA, S.; NAKAI, Y.; YOSHIDA, K., and NISHIMURA, H.: Two cases of laryngeal web. (Japanese text.) *Pract Otol Kyoto, 59:*496-500, 1966.

684. SHIPP, T.: Frequency, duration, and perceptual measures in relation to judgments of alaryngeal speech acceptability. *J Speech Hearing Res, 10:*417-27, 1967.

685. SHIPP, T.; DEATSCH, W. W., and ROSS, J. A. T.: *Pharyngoesophageal Activity in Laryngectomees.* Progress report. National Institute of Neurological Disease and Blindness. Submitted March 10, 1967.

686. SHROFF, P. D.: Carcinoma of the larynx. *J Laryng, 76:*221-28, 1962.

687. SHRYOCK, R. H.: *The Development of Modern Medicine; An Interpretation of the Social and Scientific Factors Involved.* New York, Knopf, 1947.

688. SHRYOCK, R. H.: Speech without a larynx. *Hygeia, 25:*725-53, 1947.

689. SICHEL, D., and KLOTZ, V.: Tomographies de cancer du larynx. *J Radiol Élect, 31:*11-12, 1950.

690. Siebert, T. L.; Stein, J., and Poppel, M. H.: Variations in the roentgen appearance of the "esophageal lip." *Amer J Roentgen, 81:*570-75, 1959.

691. Siegel, J. R.: Speech rehabilitation for laryngoplasty. *J Speech hearing Dis, 24:*157-8, 1959.

692. Siegel, S.: *Nonparametric Statistics: For the Behavioral Sciences.* New York, McGraw, 1956.

693. Simon, C. T.: The variability of consecutive wave lengths in vocal and instrumental sounds. *Psychol Monogr, 36:*41-83, 1927.

694. Simpson, W. L.: Treatment of cancer of the larynx with special reference to esophageal voice. *Memphis Med J, 86:*86-87, 1946.

695. Siroky, J.: Ergebnisse der Reedukation der Stimme nach der Laryngektomie. (Results of reeducation of the voice after laryngectomy.) *Z Laryng Rhinol Otol, 39:*504-12, 1960.

696. Sirtori, C.; Leonardelli, G. B., and Parolari.: Plurifocalité du cancer laryngé: Son rôle dans les récidives. (Plurifocality of laryngeal cancer: Its role in recurrences.) *J Franc Otorinolaring, 13:*549-57, 1964.

697. Skolnik, E. M.; Loewy, A., and Smoler, J.: Experiences with partial laryngopharyngectomy. *Ann Otol, 73:*417-25, 1964.

698. Skolyszewski, J.: Pooperacyjne napromienianie chorych po calkowitym wycieciu krtani. (Post-surgical irradiation of patients after radical laryngectomy. Summary.) *Otolaryng Pol, 19:*297-300, 1965.

699. Sloan, R. F. *et al.*: The application of cephalometrics to cinefluorography. *Angle Orthodont, 34:*1964.

700. Sloan, R. F. *et al.*: Radiological instrumentation in speech pathology and otology. *The Voice, J Calif, Speech Hearing Ass, 12:*1963.

701. Smirnov, A. I.: Electrocardiographic findings during esophageal and gastric surgery. *Khirurgiia (Moskva), 2:*3-15, 1955.

702. Smith, A. C.; Spalding, J. M. K.; Ardran, G. M., and Livingstone, G.: Laryngectomy in the management of severe dysphagia in nonmalignant conditions. *Lancet,   :*1094-96, 1966.

703. Smith, J. K.; Rise, E. N., and Gralnek, D. E.: Speech recovery in laryngectomized patients. *Laryngoscope, 76:*1540-46, 1966.

704. Snidecor, G. W.: *Statistical Methods.* Ames, Iowa State, 1946, p. 485.

705. Snidecor, J. C.: Los metodos de instruccion del laringectomizado en los estados unidos de America. *Acta Otorinolaring Iber Amer, 14:* 567-74, 1965.

706. Snidecor, J. C.: An objective study of phrasing in impromptu speaking and oral reading. *Speech Mono, 11:*97-104, 1944.

707. Snidecor, J. C.: Temporal aspects of breathing in superior reading and speaking performances. *Speech Mono, 22:*248-89, 1955.

708. Snidecor, J. C., and Curry, E. T.: How effectively can the laryngectomee speak? *Laryngoscope, 70:*1:62-67, 1960.

709. Snidecor, J. C., and Curry, E. T.: Temporal and pitch aspects of superior esophageal speech. *Ann Otol, 68:*623-36, 1959.

710. SNIDECOR, J. C., and ISSHIKI, N.: Air volume and air flow relationships of six male esophageal speakers. *J Speech Hearing Dis, 30:*205-16, 1965.

711. SNIDECOR, J. C., and ISSHIKI, N.: Vocal and air use characteristics of a superior male esophageal speaker. *Folia Phoniat, 17:*217-32, 1965.

712. SOBOTKOWSKI, K., and TRONCZYNSKA, J.: Anatomiczne warunki wytwo-zenia glosu przelykowego po laryngektomii. (Anatomical conditions producing esophageal voice after laryngectomy. Summary.) *Otolaryng Pol, 19:*215-20, 1965.

713. SOLIS-COHEN, J.: Diseases of the throat and nasal passage. *J Laryng, 6:* 285, 1892.

714. SOLIS-COHEN, J.: Return of the voice after laryngectomy. *JAMA, 21:*834, 1893.

715. SOM, M. L.: Surgical treatment of carcinoma of the epiglottis by lateral pharyngotomy. *Trans Amer Acad Ophth Otolaryng, 63:*28-49, 1959.

716. *Some Helpful Information to Speech Recovery After Your Laryngectomy.* Department of Otolaryngology, Cleveland Clinic.

717. SOULAS, A.: Radiocinématographic et télévision de l'ésophage; perspectives d'avenir; le temps buccopharyngien de la deglutition (présentation d'un film de Ramsey, G. H.). *Ann Otol (Paris), 73:*167-70, 1956.

718. STEINTHAL: La parole sans larynx. *Med Corresp Blatt Wurt Arztl Landesvereins, 27:*1912.

719. STERN, H.: Beiträge zur Kenntniss usw. *Z Laryng Rhinol, 12:*196, 1925.

720. STERN, H.: Das Tracheostoma als stimmgebender Apparat. *Z Hals-usw Hlk, 37:*389, 1935.

721. STERN, H.: Demonstration eines Laryngektomierten Patienten mit besonders gut modulationsfähiger Stimme. *Wien Klin Wschr, 39:* 302, 1926.

722. STERN, H.: Demonstration laryngektomierter Patienten. *Wien Med Wschr, 2:*882, 1929.

723. STERN, H.: Der Mechanismus der Sprechund Stimmbildung bei Laryngektomierten und die bei darartigen Faellen angewandte Uebungstherapie. In Denker and Kahler (Eds.): *Handb. Hals-usw. Heilk.* Berlin, Springer, 1929, vol. 5, p. 494.

724. STERN, H.: Die Funktion des Magens als Luftkessel beim Mechanismus der Sprache und Stimme Laryngektomierter. *Verh Deutsch Ges Inn Med, 35:*Kong. 90, 1923.

725. STERN, H.: Die Symptomatischen Sprachstorunger, In Gutzmann, H., Sr.: *Lehrbuch der Sprachheilkunde,* 3rd ed. Berlin, Kornfeld, 1924.

726. STERN, H.: Grundprinzipien der Sprach-u. Stimmausbildung bei laryngektomierten, nebst einem neuen Beitrag zum Machanismus der Sprach u. Stimme derartig Operierten. *Wien Klin Wschr, 33:*540, 1920.

727. STERN, H.: Kombinierter Sprechmechanismus bei einem Laryngekto-

mierten nach partieller Magenresktion. *Mschr Ohrenheilk, 66:*1173, 1932.

728. STERN, H.: Weitere Untersuchungen über den Mechanismus usw. Zentralbl. *Zbl Hals Nas Ohrenheilk, 3:*418, 1923 .

729. STETSON, R. H.: Can all laryngectomized patients be taught esophageal speech? *Trans Amer Laryng Ass, 59:*59-71, 1937.

730. STETSON, R. H.: Esophageal speech; methods of instruction after laryngectomy. *Arch Néerl Phon Exp, 13:*101, 1937.

731. STETSON, R. H.: Esophageal speech for any laryngectomized patient. *Arch Otolaryng (Chicago), 26:*132-42, 1937.

732. STETSON, R. H.: *Motor Phonetics: A Study of Speech Movements in Action,* 2nd ed. Amsterdam, North Holland, 1951.

733. STEVENS, S. S.: *Handbook of Experimental Psychology.* New York, Wiley, 1951.

734. STEVENS, S. S., and VOLKMANN, J.: The relation of pitch to frequency. *Amer J Psychol, 53:*329-53, 1940.

735. STOERK, K.: *Klinikder Krankheiten des Kehlkopfes.* Stuttgart, Ferdinand Enk, 1880, p. 546.

736. STOERK, K.: Ueber Exstipation des Larynx bei Karzinom. *Arch Laryng Rhin (Berl), 5:*22, 1896.

737. STOERK, K.: Ueber Larynxexstirpation wegen Krebs. *Wien Med Wschr, 37:*1585, 1631, 1887.

738. STOLL, B.: Psychological factors determining the success or failure of the rehabilitation program of laryngectomized patients. *Ann Otol, 67:* 550-57, 1958.

739. STORCHI, O. F., and MICHELI-PELLEGRINI, V.: Concerning the recurrent nerve innervation in the laryngectomized patient. Extract from: *Boll Mal Orecch, 77:*3-14, 1959.*

740. STORCHI, O. F., and MICHELI-PELLEGRINI, V.: A proposito del'innervazione ricorrenziale del muscolo cricofaringeo e della sua importanza nella fonazione dei laringoctomizzati. (The innervation of the cricopharyngeus muscle by the recurrent nerve and its relation with phonation in laryngectomized persons.) *Boll Mal Orecch, 77:*110-21, 1959.

741. STROTHER, C., in FROESCHELS, E.: *Twentieth Century Speech and Voice Correction.* Philadelphia, Philosophical Lib., 1948, pp. 302-12.

742. STRUBEN, W. H., and VAN GELDER, L.: Movement of the superior structures in the laryngectomized patient. *Arch Otolaryng (Chicago), 67:* 655-59, 1958.

743. STRÜBING, P.: De la parole articulée après exstirpation du larynx. *Virchow Arch Path Anat, 122:*189, 1891.

744. STRÜBING, P.: Pseudostimme nach Ausschaltung des Kehlkopfes, speciell nach Exstirpation desselben. *Deutsch Med Wschr, 14:*1061-63, 1888.

745. STRÜBING, P.: Ueber Sprachbildung nach Ausschaltung des Kehlkopfs. *Virchow Arch Path Anat., 122:*284-301, 1890.

746. Sudeck, R.: Die Pharynxsprache bie Laryngektomierten. *Deutsch Med Wschr, 48:*85, 1922.

747. Sugano, M.: Study on oesophageal speech. *J Jap Bronchooesophag Soc, 13:*135, 1962.

748. Suter, C.: Erfahrungen mit der partiellen Laryngektomie. (Results of partial laryngectomy.) *Pract Otorhinolaryngol, 23:*130-27, 1961.

749. Svane-Knudsen, V.: The substitute voice of the laryngectomized patient. *Acta Otolaryng (Stockholm), 52:*85-93, 1959.

750. Symonds, C. J.: Total laryngectomy; indications for and results of the operation. *J Laryng, 35:*257-63, 1920.

751. Symonds, C. J.: A note on the later history of 4 cases of total laryngectomy. *Lancet, 1:*652, 1920.

752. Szymanski, J.: Wyniki leczenia raka krtani chordektomia i hemilaryngectomia. (The results of chordectomy and hemilaryngectomy in cancer of the larynx.) *Otolaryng Pol, 16:*585-88, 1962.

753. Tait, V., and Tait, R. V.: Speech rehabilitation with the oral vibrator. *Speech Path Ther, 2:*64-69, 1959.

754. *Talk, 34:*Oct. 1953; *36:*Dec. 1955; *38:*Mar.-Apr. 1957.

755. Tapia, A. G.: Presentación de un laringuectomizado hablando con un sencillismo aparato artificial. *Rev Esp Laring (Madrid), 4:*49-55, 1914.

756. Tapia, A. R.: Commentary on the work of Dr. Alfonso Garibay Fernandez entitled: Emotional aspects of the laryngectomized patient. *Cir Cir, 23:*586-88, 1955.

757. Tapia, R. G.: Recuperación del laringectomizado. *Cad Cient, 4:*605, 1954.

758. Taptas, N.: Larynx artificiel extrene. *La Parole, 10:*182, 1900.

759. Taptas, N.: Un cas de laryngectomie totale pour sarcome; larynx artificiel externe. *Ann Mal Oriel Larynx, 26:*37-45, 1900.

760. Tarneaud, J.: La voix du laryngectomisé. *Ann Otolaryng (Paris), 65:*155-58, 1948.

761. Tarneaud, J.: Les maladies du larynx. *Encyclopédie Medico-Chirurgiale.* Paris, O. R. L., 1951.

762. Tarneaud, J.: *Traité pratique de Phonologie et de Phoniatrie.* Paris, Maloine, 1939.

763. Tato, J. M., Mariani, N.; DePiccoli, E. M., and Mirasov, P.: Study of the sonospectrographic characteristics of the voice in laryngectomized patients. *Acta Otolaryng (Stockholm), 44:*431-38, 1954.

764. Templeton, F. E., and Fredel, R. A.: The cricopharyngeal sphincter—a roentgenologic study. *Laryngoscope, 53:*1-12, 1943.

765. Teixeira, S. B.: Pseudo-voz dos laringectomizados. *Arch Brasil Med, 41:*21-26, 1951.

766. Terracol, J.: *Les Maladies de L'oesophage.* Paris, Masson, 1951.

767. Tetu, I.; Arteni, V.; Ghim-Peteanu, M.; Graciun, E.; Dimitriu, A. V.; Bernea, A., and Danciulescu, V.: Consideratii in legatura cu roentgenterapia de contact in cancerul laringian. (On contact roentgeno-

therapy in the cancer of the larynx.) *Otorinolaryng Ruman, 9:*303-09, 1964.

768. TEZEL, E. B.: Automatic return of speech after laryngectomy for cancer. *Turk Tip Cem Mec, 5:*31, 1939.

769. The patient with carcinoma of the larynx. Somatopsychic Conference of the University of Illinois College of Medicine. *GP, 11:*84-93, 1955.

770. THOMAS, H. M., III.: Esophageal speech. *Med Times, 87:*454-61, 1959.

771. THOMPSON, ST. CLAIR: *Disease of the Nose and Throat.* London, Cassell & Co., 1955, p. 619.

772. THOMPSON, ST. CLAIR: History of cancer of the larynx. *J Laryng, 54:* 61-87, 1939.

773. THORNVAL, A.: The result of laryngectomies performed during the period from 1928 to 1945. *Acta Otolaryng (Stockholm), 34:*331, 1946.

774. TIKOFSKY, R. S.: A comparison of the intelligibility of esophageal and normal speakers. *Folia phoniat, 17:*19-32, 1965.

775. TIKOFSKY, RITA P.; GLATTKE, T. J., and PERRY, P. S.: Listener Identification of Esophageal Production of Voiced and Voiceless Consonants. ASHA Convention Report, San Francisco, 1964.

776. TORP, I. M.: X-rays for the voice instructor. *Radiography, 20:*238:210-13, 1954.

777. TRAVIS, L. E.: *Handbook of Speech Pathology.* New York, Appleton, 1957.

778. TSUKERBERG, L. I.: Respiratory function in patients after laryngectomy. *Vestn Otorinolaring, 20:*91-95, 1958.

779. TUCKER, G.: Diagnosis and treatment of cancer of the larynx. *JAMA, 149:*119-21, 1952.

780. ULLMANN, E. V.: Über Beziehungen des Riechvermögens zum Kehlkopf, zugleich ein Beitrag zur Physiol. des Riechaktes. *Z Hals Nas Ohrenheilk, 6:*570, 1923.

781. U.S. Department of Health, Education and Welfare: *Cancer of the Larynx.* Public Health Service Publication No. 1294, 1965.

782. VAHERI, E.: Results on laryngectomy in one hundred cases of cancer of the larynx. *Acta Otolaryng (Stockholm), 46:*439-45, 1956.

783. VALLANCIEN, B., and DINVILLE, C.: Application de la radiocinémonométrie à l'etude de la voix oesophagienne. (Application of radiocinemanometry to the study of esophageal voice.) *J Franc Otorinolaring, 12:*223-26, 1963.

784. VALLANCIEN, B.; DINVILLE, C.; BESANCON, F.; CHERIGIE, E.; LABAYLE, J., and LE HUCHIE, F.: La voix oesophagienne. (Esophageal voice.) *J Franc Otorinolaring, 15:*427-29, 1966.

785. VANDOR, F.: Roentgen studies of the pseudoglottis in laryngectomized patients. *Fortschr Roentgenstr, 82:*618-25, 1955.

786. VILAR-SANCHO ALTET, B.: Latest reflections on laryngectomy. *Acta Otorinolaring Iber Amer, 9:*367-96, 1958.

787. VOKOUN, F. J.: Resection of the larynx without loss of the voice. *Milit Surg, 69:*617, 1931.

788. VON LEDEN, H.: The electronic synchon-stroboscope. *Ann Otol, 70:*1-13, 1961.

789. VON LEDEN, H.: The mechznism of phonation. *Arch Otolaryng (Chicago), 74:*660-76, 1961.

790. VOORHOEVE, N.: Der Magan als vikariierender Luftkessel nach Laryngektomie. *Acta Radiol (Stockholm), 7:*587-94, 1926.

791. VRTICKA, K., and PETRIK, M.: Rehabilitation of laryngectomized patients by substitute esophageal speech and electronic vocal aids. *Cesk Otolaryng, 16:*19-25, 1967.

792. VRTICKA, K., and SVOBODA, M.: A clinical and x-ray study of 100 laryngectomized speakers. *Folia Phoniat, 13:*174-86, 1961.

793. VRTICKA, K., and SVOBODA, M.: Time changes in the x-ray picture of the hypopharynx, pseudoglottis, and esophagus in the course of vocal rehabilitation in 70 laryngectomized speakers. *Folia Phoniat, 15:* 1-12, 1963.

794. WALDROP, W. F.: Rehabilitation of the laryngectomized patient. *Nebraska Med J, 39:*419-22, 1954.

795. WALDROP, W. F., and GOULD, M. A.: *Your New Voice.* Chicago Amer Cancer Society, (Illinois Division) Inc., 1956.

796. WALDROP, W. F., and TOHT, A. E.: Analysis of Vowels of Laryngectomized Speakers. ASHA Convention Report, 1958.

797. WALL, C. B.: Irritating angel: M. Doehler, teacher of esophageal speech. *Reader's Digest, 74:*69-73, 1959.

798. WALLACH, G. C.: An Experimental Comparison of the Two Major Types of Electrolarynges from the Standpoint of Intelligibility and Subjective Reaction of the Listener. Unpublished M.A. thesis, University of Arizona, 1960.

799. WARD, P. H.; FREDRICKSON, J. M.; STRADJORD, N. M., and VALVASSORI, G. E.: Laryngeal and pharyngeal pouches. Surgical approach and the use of cinefluorographic and other radiologic techniques as diagnostic aids. *Laryngoscope,* 564-82, 1963.

800. WATSON, P. H.: (Cited by Stevenson, R. S., and Guthrie, D.) *History of Otolaryngology.* Baltimore, Williams and Wilkins, 1949, p. 85.

801. WEBB, M. W., and IRVING, R. W.: Psychologic and anamnestic patterns characteristic of laryngectomees; relation to speech rehabilitation. *J Amer Geriat Soc, 12:*303-22, 1964.

802. WEERSMA, P.: Spraak zonder larynx. *Nederl T Geneesk, 84:*3070, 1940.

803. WEGEL, R. L.: Mechanics of larynx, natural and artificial. *Trans Amer Laryng Rhin Otol Soc, 36:*319-20, 1930.

804. WEIHA, H.: Effect of movement of adjoining organs on production of esophageal speech. *Arch Ohr Nas Kehlkopfheilk, 173:*529-33, 1958.*

805. WEISS, D., and GRÜNBERG, M.: Roentgenography of normal phonation

and that of laryngectomized patients. *Bull Soc Belge Otol Lar Rhin,* pp. 373-83, 1939.

806. WELDER, H. W., and SCHWAB, W.: X-ray appearance of the hypopharynx after laryngectomy. *Arch Ohr Nas Kehlkopfheilk, 168:*8-18, 1955.

807. WEPMAN, J. M.; MACGAHAN, J. A.; RICHARD, J. C., and SKELTON, N. W.: The objective measurement of progressive esophageal speech development. *J Speech Hearing Dis, 18:*249-50, 1953.

808. WESSELY, V. E.: Verschlussplastik eines laryngotracheostomas mit Wiederherstellung der normalen Sprechstimme. *Mschr Ohrenheilk, 78:* 1145, 1936.

809. WEST, R. W.; KENNEDY, L.; CARR, A., with BACKUS, O. L.: *The Rehabilitation of Speech.* New York, Harper, 1947.

810. WEST, R. W.; ANSBERRY, M., and CARR, A.: *The Rehabilitation of Speech.* New York, Harper, 1957.

811. WETHERHILL: Retour de la voix apres une laryngectomie totale. *Ann Mal Oreil Larynx,* p. 10, 1894.

812. WHITE, WILLARD: Speech rehabilitation following laryngectomy; the role of the therapist. *Talk, 36:*9-10, 13, 1955.

813. WHITE, W. C.: Analysis of the Rate and Intensity of Laryngectomized vs. Normal Speakers Reading Under Conditions of Side-tone Delay. Unpublished M.A. thesis, The Ohio State University, 1962.

814. WILDENBERG, VAN DEN: What rehabilitation can do. Speech without a larynx. *Hosp Progr, 31:*237-41, 1950.

815. WILDENBERG, VAN DEN: La laryngectomie totale chez un octogénaire. *Acta Otorhinolaryng (Belg), 5:*362, 1951.

816. WINCKEL, Elektroakustiche Untersuchungen. *Folia phoniat (Basel), 4:* 1952.

817. WINTERSTEEN, L. L.: Speech rehabilitation of the laryngectomized person. *Arch Phys Med Rehab, 44:*454-56, 1963.

818. WOLFF, J.: Ueber Verbesserungen am kuenstlichen Kehlkopf usw. *Arch Klin Chir, 45:*237, 1892.

819. WOLFF, J.: Ueber den kuenstlichen Kehlkopf und die Pseudo-Stimme. *Berl Klin Wschr, 30:*1009, 1893.

820. WOODMAN, D., and KASTEIN, S.: Voice rehabilitation via laryngeal surgery and speech therapy. *New York J Med, 57:*60-62, 1957.

821. WOOKEY, H.: The treatment of lesions of the hypopharynx and upper esophagus. *Brit J Surg, 35:*251-56, 1948.

822. WRIGHT, E. S.: Diagnosis and treatment of cancer of the larynx. *Ann Otol, 51:*228, 1942.

823. WRIGHT, J. W.: *A History of Laryngology and Rhinogology.* Philadelphia, Lea & F, 1914.

824. WYNDER, E. L.; BROSS, I. J., and DAY, E.: Epidemiological approach to the etiology of cancer of the larynx. *JAMA, 160:*1384, 1956.

825. YANAGIHARA, N.: Significance of harmonic changes and noise components in hoarseness. *J Speech Hearing Res, 10:*531-41, 1967.

826. ZAKRZEWSKI, A.: Tluszczak krtani (o lokalizacji podglosniowej.) (Lipoma of the larynx.) Summary. *Otolaryn Pol, 19:*131, 1965.

827. ZAKRZEWSKI, A., and DURSKA-ZAKRZEWSKA, A.: W sprawie postepowania w otwartym poprzecznym rozerwaniu krtani. (Concerning the management in the open, transverse tearing of the larynx.) *Otolaryng Pol, 19:*181-86, 1965.

828. ZAKRZEWSKI, A.; DURSKA-ZAKRZEWSKA, A., and WOJTOWICZ, J.: O postepowaniu w calkowitym zarosnieciu górnego odcinka tchawicy i krtani w jej czesci podglosniowej. (On the management in complete obliteration of the upper part of the trachea and larynx in its subgottic part. Summary.) *Otolaryng Pol, 19:*307, 1965.

829. ZAPF, R.: Ueber die Bildung der Sprache und Stimme nach Laryngektomie. Dissertation, Hamburg, 1923.

830. ZERBA, L., and BORGO, M.: Studio istomorfologico sulla neoseudocorda dopo exeresi della corda vocale. (Histoligic study of the neopseudocord after excision of the vocal cord.) *Arch Ital Otol, 76:*89-101, 1965.

831. ZIMONT, D. I.: Present state of the problem of therapy of laryngeal cancer. *Vestn Otorinolaring, 17:*3-12, 1955.

832. ZINN, W. F.: Laryngectomy. *Trans Amer Laryng Rhinol Otol Soc, 39:* 471, 1933.

833. ZUKERBERG, L. I.: The capacity for work after laryngectomy for cancer. (Russian text.) *Vop Onkol, 6:*33-40, 1960.

*These translations will be available from S. L. A. Translations Center, The John Crerar Library, 86 East Randolph Street, Chicago 1, Illinois.

Appendix

Directory of Sources of Supply for Items of Benefit to Laryngectomees*

Note: The International Association of Laryngectomees respects the ethical practices code of the medical profession in every way. Therefore, we publish this directory simply as a service to laryngectomees everywhere, and do not recommend any item in particular. We urge that you do not use this directory in connection with a commercial venture of any kind. All particulars must be obtained directly from the source of supply.

TRACHEA TUBES, OBTURATORS
Your doctor, surgeon, or local surgical supply house.
BIBS, AIR FILTERS (knitted, crocheted, gauze)
Your local Lost Chord Club
New York Anamilo Club, 61 Irving Place, New York, N.Y. 10003.
(For instructions for crocheting)
IAL Office, 219 E. 42nd St. New York, N. Y. 10017.
(For instructions for making nylon bib)
STOMA SCREEN
Vincent C. Hozier, 12012 Herbert St. Los Angeles, Cal. 90066.
Kenneth Lockwood, 10916 Thornton, Cleveland, Ohio 44125.
John McClear, 61 Irving Place, New York, N. Y. 10003.
ASPIRATORS (heavy-duty or portable)
Your local office of the American Cancer Society (for Free Loan, if available) .
Your local surgical supply house.
SHOWER COLLARS
C. L. Sheldon, 311 School St., Watertown, Mass. 02172.
HOME HUMIDIFIERS
Electric type: Your local electric appliance dealer.
Permanent type: Your local plumbing firm (for installation on your heating plant) .

---

*Published with the permission of IAL.

EMERGENCY

(Bracelet) — Medic-Alert Foundation, 1030 Sierra Dr., Turlock, Cal. 95380.

(Pocket Card) — IAL Office, 219 E. 42nd St., New York 17, N. Y.

(Auto Sticker) IAL Treasurer Frank Wingo, 813 Taylorville Blvd., Taylorville, Ill.

Civil Defense Office, your city or state.

MANUALS OF INSTRUCTION IN POST-LARYNGECTOMY SPEECH

Esophageal Speech by Doehler
American Cancer Society, 138 Newbury St., Boston Mass.

Your New Voice by Waldrop and Gould
American Cancer Society, your local office.

How To Speak Again by Hyman and Keller
Dr. M. Hyman, Bowling Green State Univ., Bowling Green, Ohio. (Also in Spanish language)

PHONOGRAPH RECORDS FOR POST LARYNGECTOMY SPEECH INSTRUCTION

Mrs. Paul A. Doehler, 243 Charles St., Boston, Mass.

Dr. M. Hyman, Bowling Green State Univ., Bowling Green, Ohio.

ARTIFICIAL LARYNGES

Aurex Corp., 315 W. Adams St., Chicago, Ill.

Kett Engineering Co., 920 Santa Monica Blvd., Santa Monica, Cal.

Rand Development Corp., 12720 Lake Shore Blvd., Cleveland 8, Ohio.

Bell Telephone Co., your local office.

(Available in foreign countries through World Health Organization of the United Nations. Contact health or foreign minister.)

AMPLIFIERS FOR WEAK VOICES

Rand Development Corp., 12720 Lake Shore Blvd., Cleveland 8, Ohio.

Brenkert & Deming, Box 47, Royal Oak, Mich. 48068.

IAL Office, 219 E. 42nd St., New York, N. Y. 10017.

(Do-it-yourself model plans)

TAPE RECORDERS

Your local dealer in electric appliances and sound reproduction.

PUBLICATIONS OF THE IAL

IAL NEWS.

Published bimonthly — free.

Laryngectomees' Manual — IAL program for local chapters. Basic organization and program. 22 pages.

Directory.

Published annually. Includes Officers, Directors, Advisors, and committees; as well as affiliated clubs, their officers, meeting dates, places and times; and facilities for speech instructions. 60 pages.

First-aid for Laryngectomees (pamphlet).

Gives special instructions for first-aid to laryngectomees. For distribution to all kinds of public safety officials. Available through your local office of the American Cancer Society or local Lost Chord Club. (Code #3015). 10 pages. (*Instructor's Manual* — Lost Chords of New Jersey, 843 E. 27th St., Paterson, New Jersey.)

Bibliography on Rehabilitation of Laryngectomees.

Lists articles of interest to members of the medical profession and postlaryngectomy speech instructors. Revised, January 1967. 26 pages.

Helping Words (pamphlet).

For the new patient. Gently explains what has happened and how the patient can live a normal life in the future. For distribution by doctors and competent laryngectomees. Available through your local office of the American Cancer Society or local Lost Chord Club. (#4511). 22 pages.

Rehabilitating Laryngectomees (pamphlet).

For use as a give-away piece at lectures, exhibits, and for new patients. Available through your local office of the American Cancer Society (#4506). 10 pages.

Laryngectomees at Work (pamphlet).

A direct appeal to employers in order to encourage them to employ or reemploy laryngectomees. (#4519) 8 pages.

Reprints

The IAL attempts to obtain reprints of articles of interest to laryngectomees which appear in the national periodicals and leading newspapers. Also, addresses and proceedings of annual meetings..

Other Publications.

Your Latest Challenge — That New Voice. Published by Florida Laryngectomee Ass'n., 617 Flagler Bldg., Tampa 2, Fla.

You Can Speak Again. Published by Detroit Anamilo Club, 4811 John R St., Detroit, Mich.

EXHIBITS

"Esophageal Speech Following Laryngectomy" (10' x 3') This is a full-sized exhibit for professional meetings, etc.

"Esophageal Speech Following Laryngectomy" (3' x 5') Copy of same exhibit as above. Can be used at smaller meetings.

FILMS

Code # HN-2: *Total Laryngectomy for Carcinoma.* D. R. Weaver, M.D. 3 reels, 1200 ft., 35 minutes, color, silent. 1948. For professional use only.

HN-6: *Organic Disorders of the Larynx.* Paul H. Holinger, M.D. 1 reel, 800 ft., 22 minutes, color, silent. 1947. For professional use only.

3424: *Head and Neck Cancer.* Presented by Martin Hayes, M.D. Kinescope of closed-circuit TV film. 16 mm, 45 minutes, color, sound. For professional use only.

3440: *Cancer Detection.* Presented by Emerson Day, M.D. Kinescope of closed-circuit TV film. 16 mm, color, sound, *38 minute.* For professional use only.

The above-listed films should be ordered from the Medical Audio-Visual Institute of the Association of American Medical Colleges at 2530 Ridge Avenue, Evanston, Illinois. A fee of $5.00 is charged for the loan of each film to cover shipping and handling costs.

Code # 55: *New Voices.* Use of postlaryngectomy voice (Cleveland Speech & Hearing Center). 1 reel, 800 ft., 20 minutes, black-and-white or color, sound. 1948.

57: *Rehabilitation of Laryngectomized Patient* (We Speak Again). Leroy A. Schall, M.D., 1 reel, 800 ft., 22 minutes, color, sound. 1949.

58: *Speech after Laryngectomy.* Syracuse University — Commercial Motion Pictures, 1480 Salt Springs Road, Syracuse, N. Y. 1 reel, 800 ft., 22 minutes, color, sound. 1956.

16: *The Irritating Angel.* Kinescope of TV program 4/26/59. 16 mm, black-and-white, sound, $28\frac{1}{2}$ minutes.

— *Never Alone.* The American Cancer Society, including scenes about laryngectomees. 16 mm, black-and-white (also 35 mm) 28 minutes, sound. (Also, short version, *I Ate A Peach.*)

— *Cry Out in Silence.* Kinescope of "Alcoa Premiere" TV program 5/15/62. 16 mm, black-and-white, sound, $28\frac{1}{2}$ minutes.

81: *A Second Voice.* A new IAL film about total rehabilitation of the laryngectomee. 16 mm, sound, color, 14 minutes.

— *Alaryngeal Speech.* W. M. Diedrich, Ph.D. Demonstrates the teaching of postlaryngectomy speech to a new patient. 16 mm, black-and-white, sound, 20 minutes. Department of Medical Communications, University of Kansas Medical Center, Kansas City, Kansas 66103.

— *To Speak Again.* 8 mm Fairchild Cartridge. Primarily for bedside use in the hospital.

The exhibits and the films listed just above should be ordered through your local office or state Division of the American Cancer Society.

SLIDES

First Aid For Laryngectomees. Slide series produced by Indiana State Police. Running commentary or script available from IAL First Aid Committee, Mrs. Frances Gesner, 843 East 27th St., Paterson, New Jersey (free). Slide set costs approximately $10.00. Write the H. Leiber Company, 440 North Capitol Avenue, Indianapolis, Indiana. 28 slides, 35 mm.

Index

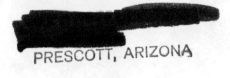

PRESCOTT, ARIZONA